THE ART OF SLOWING DOWN

First published as *Slow* in 2018

Text and picture research by Anna Martin

Additional text by Abi McMahon

An Hachette UK Company
www.hachette.co.uk

Vie Books, an imprint of Summersdale Publishers
Part of Octopus Publishing Group Limited
Carmelite House
50 Victoria Embankment
LONDON
EC4Y 0DZ
UK

www.summersdale.com

This FSC® label means that materials used for the product have been responsibly sourced

MIX
Paper | Supporting responsible forestry
FSC www.fsc.org FSC® C016973

The authorized representative in the EEA is Hachette Ireland, 8 Castlecourt Centre, Dublin 15, D15 XTP3, Ireland (email: info@hbgi.ie)

Printed and bound in China

ISBN: 978-1-83799-637-7

- THE ART OF -
SLOWING DOWN

How to Find Peace and Purpose in a Hectic World

JO PETERS

vie

CONTENTS

INTRODUCTION

It seems today that we have reached the stage of turning every moment into some sort of race. We rush to work, we rush to make dinner, we rush to get the children organized, we rush our correspondence and social interactions… where will it end? It's no wonder that many of us are made breathless by our everyday lives and want to somehow step off the treadmill. Slow living is just that – a chance to stop the idea that being busy is the be-all and end-all, to start paying attention to the important things in life, and to slow down to a pace that is right for you.

Living slowly is a stepping stone to happiness and good health, because when we live at a slower pace, we are more in the moment and able to immerse ourselves in what we are doing and take the full pleasure from it. Taking the slow lane means fewer mistakes are made, and it offers us the opportunity to be more considered in our actions. In terms of health, slowing down calms our breathing and reduces stress. There is the added benefit of building stronger relationships with friends and loved ones by taking the time to connect with each other.

Slow isn't about low efficiency or giving up your job or being idle. It's about creating balance and allocating pockets of time to plan, to think, to reflect, to observe, and to give focus to what's important – to do things better instead of faster and in turn to become more productive.

How different would your life be if you weren't whirling from one thing to the next, trying to keep the plates spinning in the air? *The Art of Slowing Down* gives you the tools to do just that – we set out ways to streamline your life and make it simpler, more efficient and more productive by doing things at the right speed – the rest is up to you.

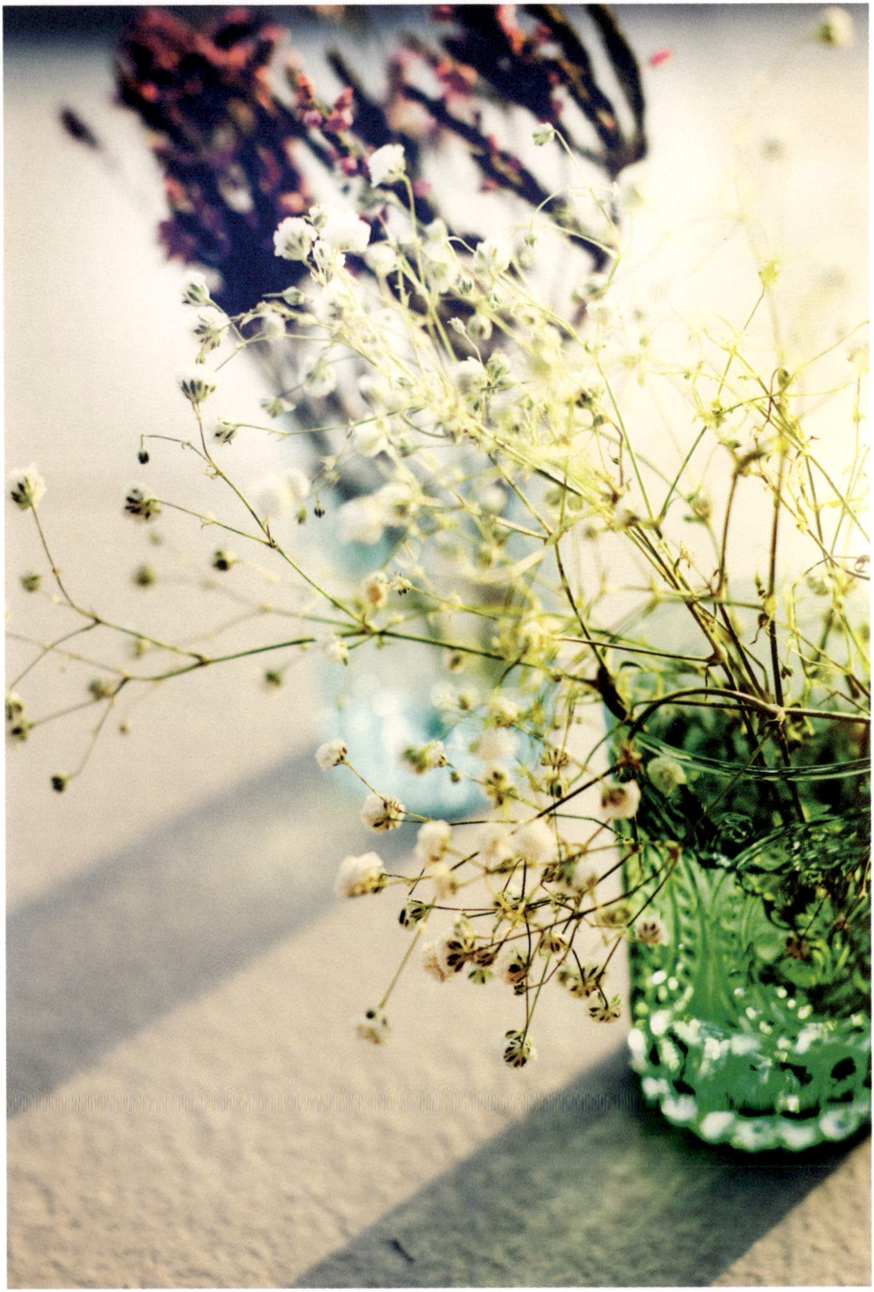

THE ORIGINS OF THE *slow movement*

The slow movement began with the creation of the slow food movement in 1986, after a man named Carlo Petrini protested against the approval of a fast food restaurant in the Piazza di Spagna, in the heart of Rome. The slow food movement promotes the principles of organic, non-processed foods where the chain from farm to table has a minimal impact on the environment.

The concept of "slow" has since filtered down into other parts of modern society, such as slow parenting and slow cities, culminating in the formation of the Norway-based World Institute of Slowness in 1999 by Geir Berthelsen, which aims to teach the world the ways of slow living.

Another notable advocate of slow living is Carl Honoré, who, in his 2004 book, *In Praise of Slow*, explored how slow living could be applied and maintained, particularly in a business environment.

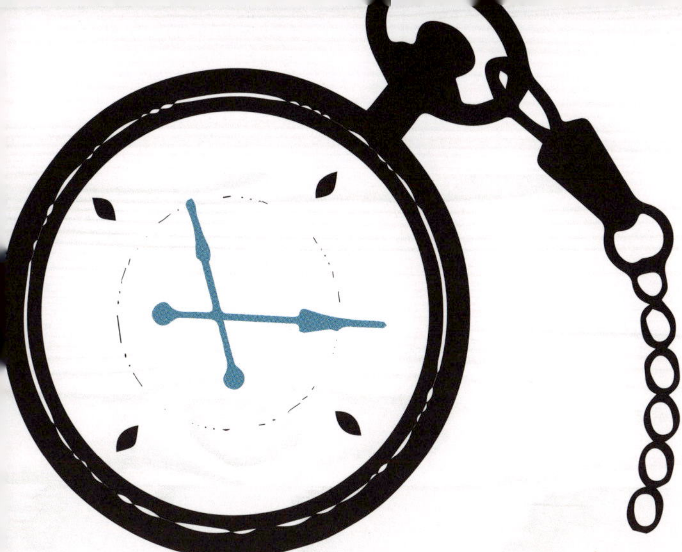

Why be fast when you can be slow?

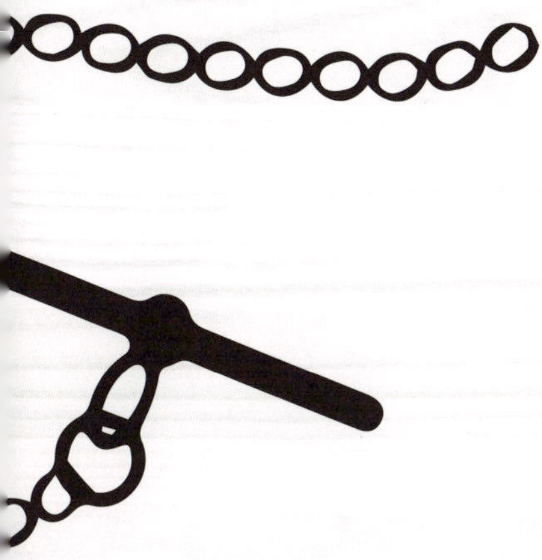

GEIR BERTHELSEN, FOUNDER OF
THE WORLD INSTITUTE OF SLOWNESS

SLOW HEALTH AND WELL-BEING

HOW TO SLOW DOWN TIME

This may seem like a tall order, but there are many ways to slow down – this section is all about discovering a slow ritual that works for you.

MINDFULNESS – CELEBRATE THE MOMENT

Maintaining a mindful attitude is a very positive way of slowing down time. Mindfulness is about focusing on the magic of the present moment. Rather than fretting about the past or worrying about the future, the aim is to experience life as it unfolds, moment by moment. This simple practice is immensely powerful and an effective tool for slowing down to a more comfortable pace. As we rush through our lives, mindfulness encourages us to stop constantly striving for something new or better and to embrace acceptance and gratitude. Many of us rush through our daily routines on autopilot, barely noticing what we are doing. An easy way to focus your attention on the present moment is to concentrate on simple tasks. For instance, make your bed with 100 per cent focus and attention each morning so you create a calm transition from bedroom and sleep to the outside world and the rest of your day. You might also find it useful to sit quietly for a few minutes in the morning so that you can calmly contemplate the day ahead, instead of rushing straight into your day's activities, or to embrace your time in the shower, taking a moment to think about the running water washing away sleep, energizing you for the rest of the day.

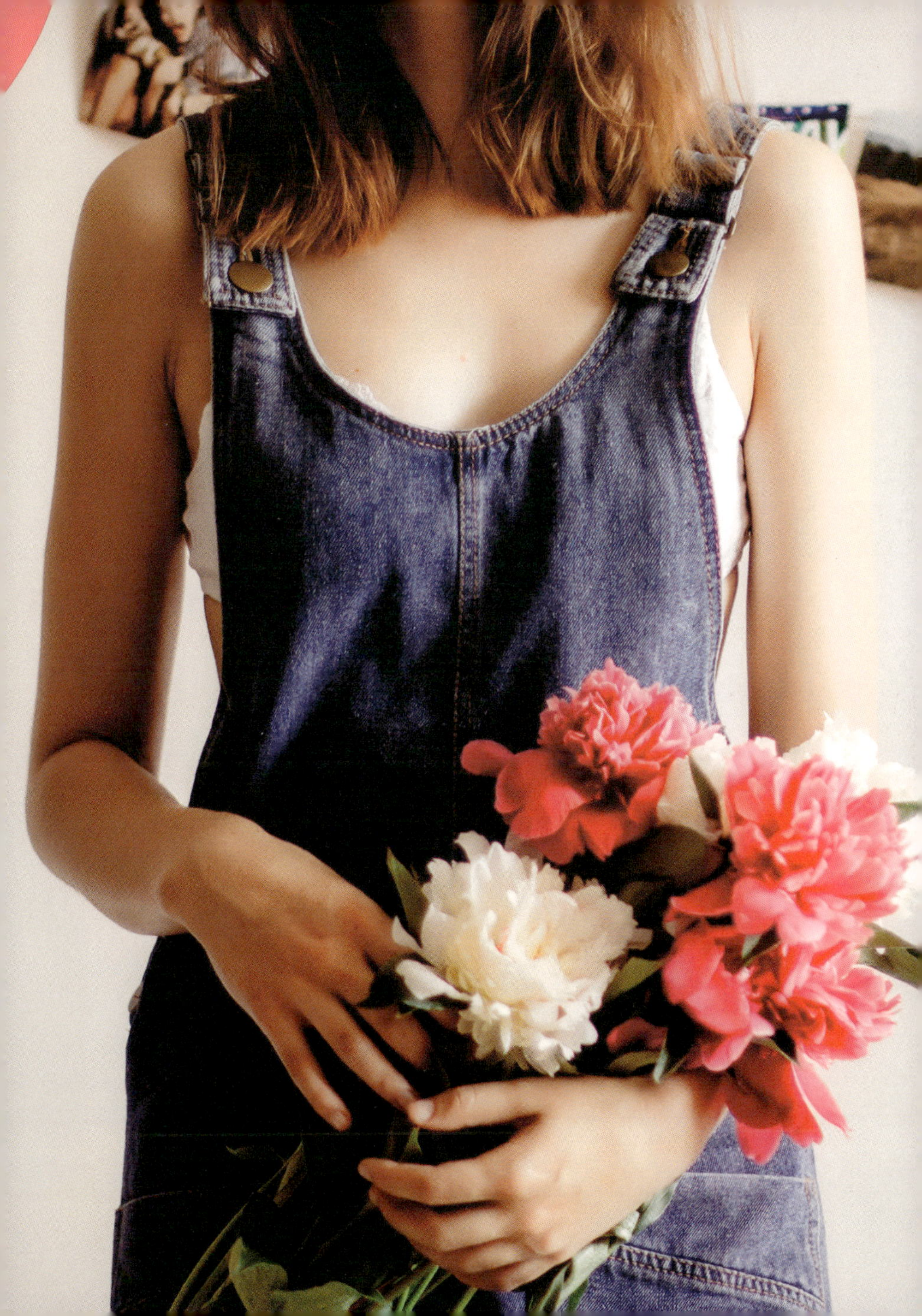

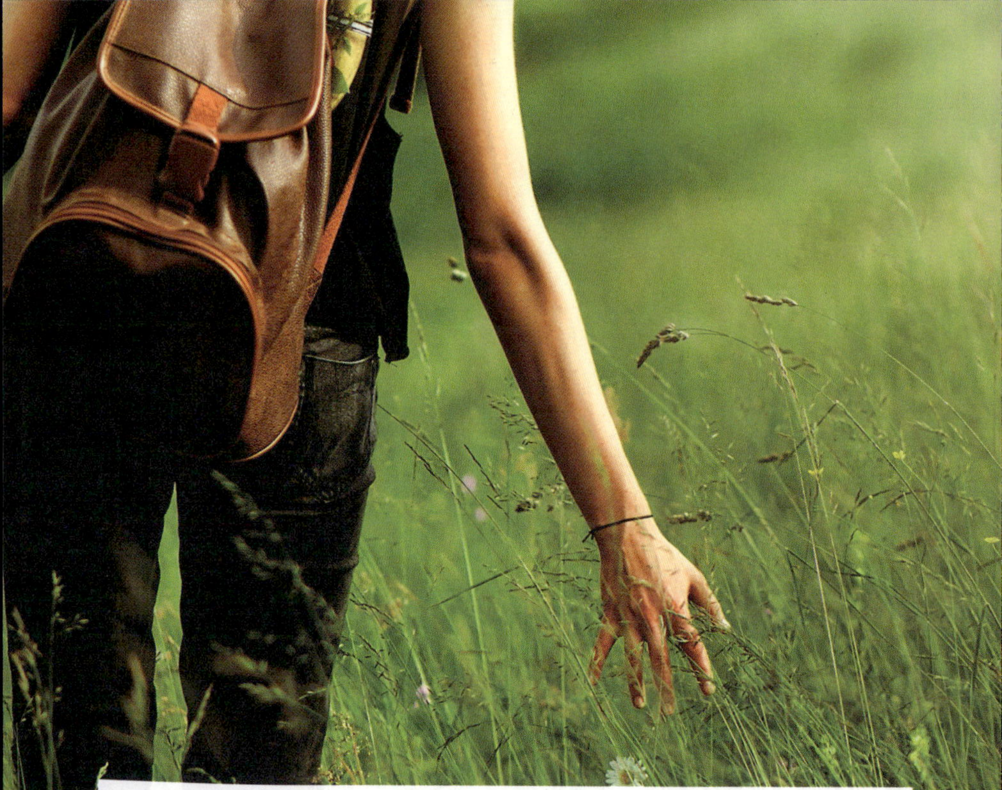

Reconnect with your body using breathing exercises

Slow, deep breathing reoxygenates the body, which slows our heartbeat and stabilizes blood pressure. Try this exercise for instant calm. This can be done at any time of the day, whether before bed, first thing in the morning or at your desk in the office. The practice is simple: close your eyes and focus on your breath. Think only about your breath and the way it feels coming into your body and then out. Once you are fully aware of your breathing, try taking deeper breaths, breathing in for a count of six and then out for a count of six. Stay focused on your breath for 5 minutes. Integrating this exercise into your daily routine will help you on your way to feeling more relaxed.

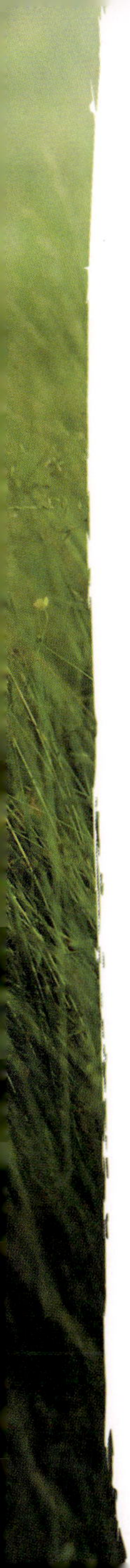

DO LESS, NOTICE MORE

Instead of cramming as much as possible into your day, do less and do it more slowly, more fully and with more concentration. Take the time to immerse yourself fully in whatever activity you're doing, whether you're cooking supper or chatting to a friend, even for the less fun activities like cleaning the dishes. You should find your experiences relaxing and fulfilling when you're not rushing through them.

STAY GROUNDED

The next time you find yourself rushing – it could be when you're on an errand or whizzing round the supermarket to get the evening meal – focus your awareness on your feet. Try to slow down your pace and feel your feet connecting you with the ground. How does it feel? Warm, cold, hard, uneven or even soft? Thinking about something as simple as the ground beneath your feet will help you to gain a sense of balance and perspective, and most importantly, slow you down.

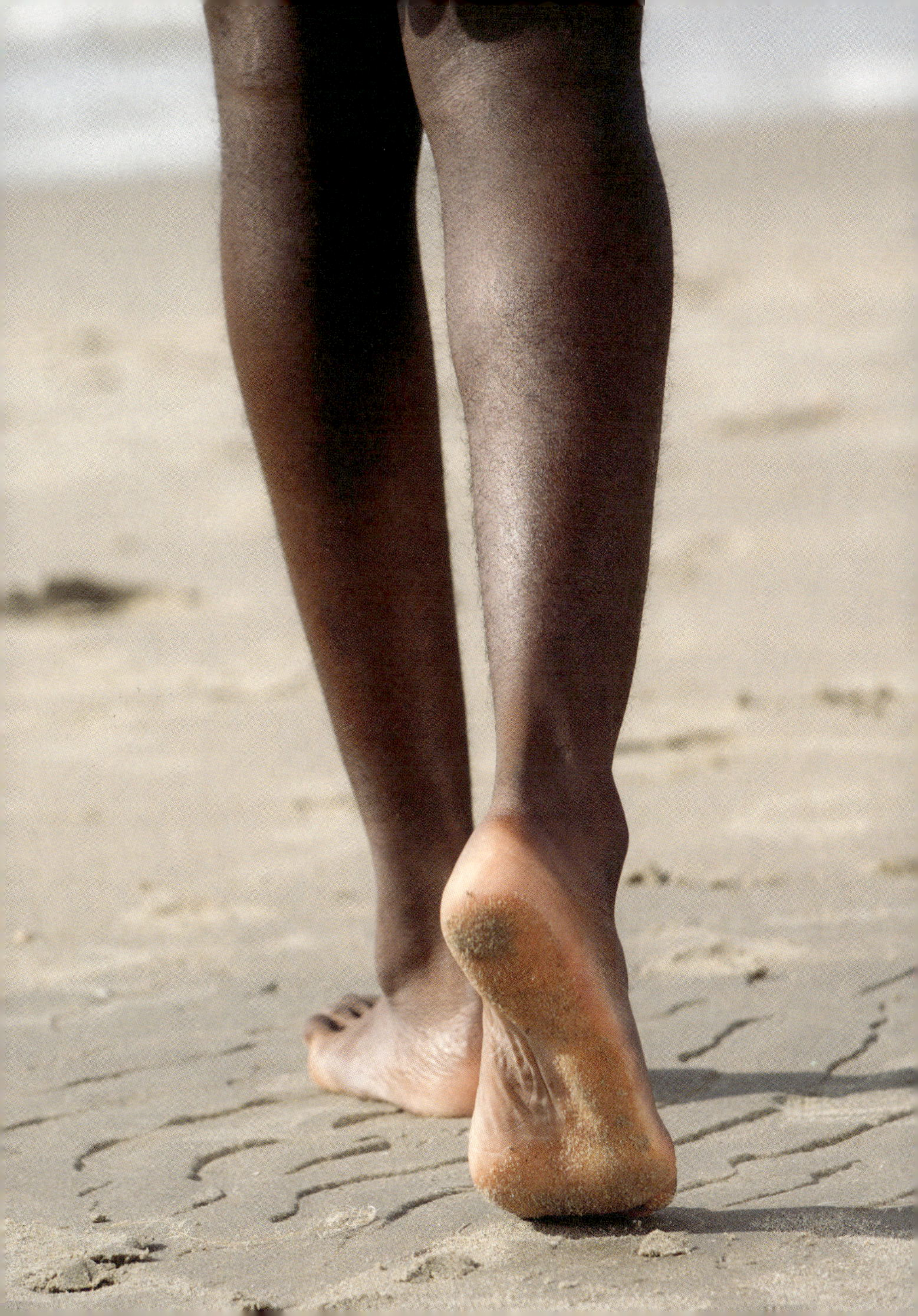

FIND YOUR SLOW RITUAL

Make time for slow hobbies. These needn't be particularly productive, but should be about savouring the time and immersing yourself in one activity without distraction purely for your own enjoyment. Channelling your energy into one slow activity will clear your head and help you to refocus, much like mindfulness, and will teach you patience and how to have a more considered approach to every aspect of your life. It's also about rediscovering a playful side that may have diminished since becoming a busy adult. Allow your slow ritual to become your personal brake and enjoy this calmer pace. Read on for some ideas to try.

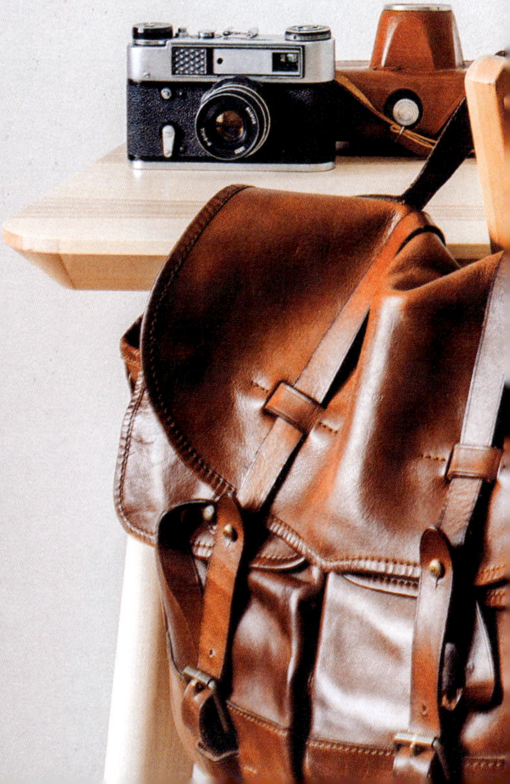

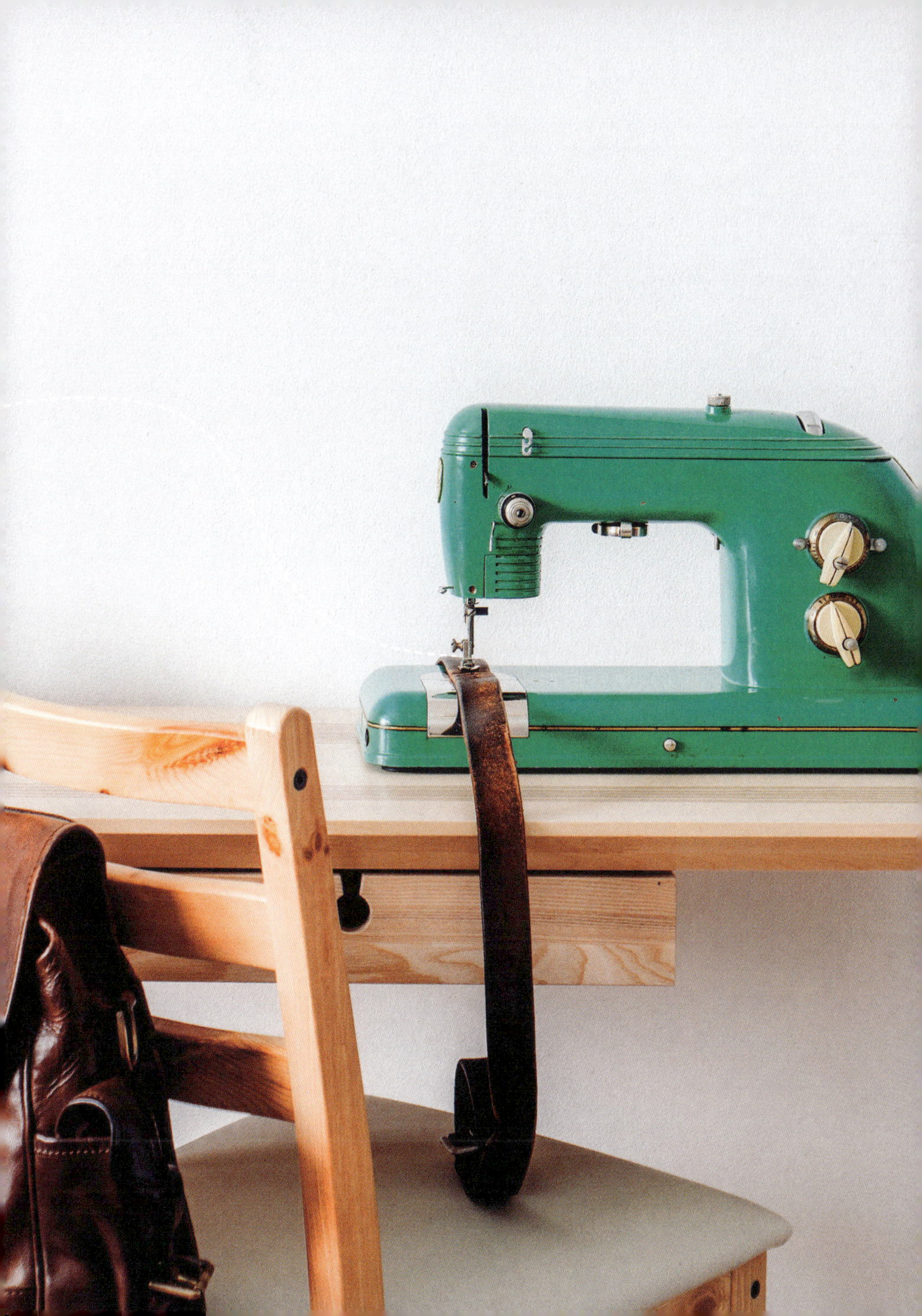

Handwriting

Get creative by stepping away from the computer and treating yourself to good, old-fashioned pen and ink – inky fingers optional (but a distinct possibility!). Not having an undo button when you are putting your thoughts on paper takes a while to get used to, but you'll find that you will work at a more considered pace and you won't suffer the ill effects of staring at a screen for extended periods.

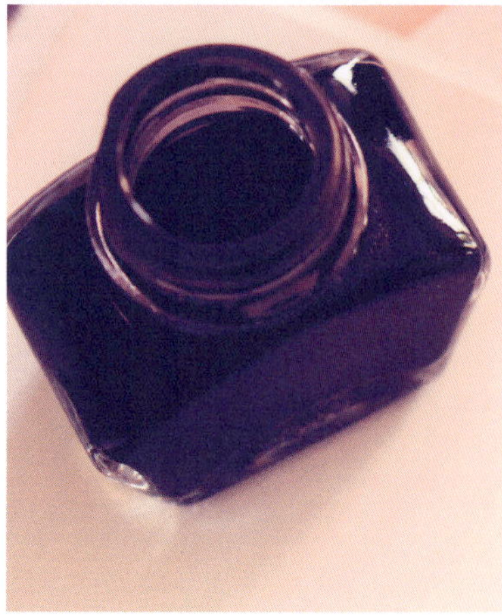

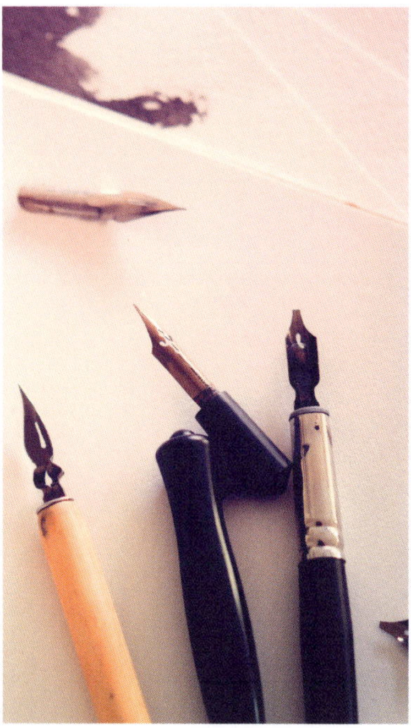

The end result needn't be a masterpiece – play with words; perhaps write a poem with two words per line, a letter to someone, or a diary entry. Carefully craft every sentence or stanza and consider every syllable – that's the wonder of handwriting as you're forced to slow down. There are many benefits to writing in longhand; according to a study by Indiana University, it stimulates neural activity in the brain which has a similar effect to meditation. It also keeps your brain sharp and may even make us more positive as well as having a healing effect. According to a study in New Zealand, those who wrote about their thoughts on paper after a traumatic event or surgery were found to heal more quickly.

Painting, drawing and colouring in

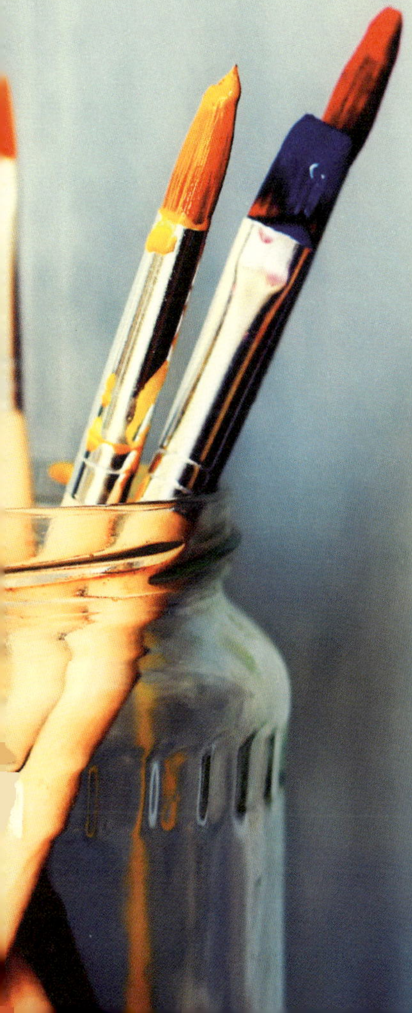

Get your paints out – swirl your brushes in the paints and play with colour. This can be a wonderful meditative process. It's important not to worry about the quality of your work but to take pleasure in creating.

There's a reason why colouring books are so popular. Colouring is proven to have the same health benefits as meditation, including reducing anxiety levels and having a restorative effect. This is because colouring in allows the brain to switch off peripheral thoughts and focus on one activity. It is a comfortable form of creative expression as it has boundaries with shapes to colour. A study by psychologists at the University of Otago in New Zealand concluded that colouring in for as little as 10 minutes a day reduced symptoms of depression and anxiety and was considered a worthwhile self-help tool when monitoring low-level incidences of these mental health conditions.

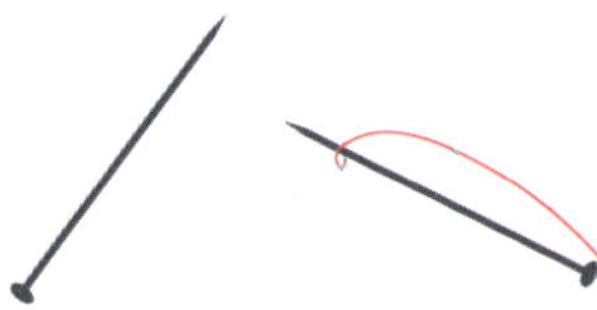

Knitting

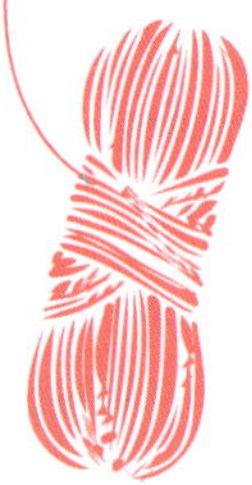

Knitting is another practice that is all-encompassing – if you want to avoid dropping stitches. Take pleasure in sourcing the wool – consider the colour and texture – and enjoy the calming, rhythmic click-click of the needles as you watch your knitting grow before your eyes. The repetition of carrying out the same steps over and over is a lesson in enjoying the process of something, rather than racing to finish. The other benefit of knitting, or indeed sewing or crochet, is that it's a portable slow hobby, which can be done when you are on a bus or train – far more therapeutic than zoning out on social media. Knitting is simple once you get started; try using an online tutorial.

PUZZLES

Crosswords, Sudoku, word searches, jigsaws – all of these puzzles are a great way to slow down and focus on one task as well as providing a sense of accomplishment. They are also great for stimulating your brain and are proven to help you stay mentally sharp as well as delaying symptoms of dementia in later life.

Try this slow word search for size.

B A T K S A T E L G N I S A S I O C

A G O A F N L E A O A I L O E M Q I

A X A H J I W Z S D A T O G D E A R

E A M A C M A X E A E U W A F M K J

M A W I T I O T R R E S A R K D E F

U V E S N E R A A D R O A A U A R D

N I T U G D A C R U Y H A G S F L O

A J H E R Q F T C N E D T L A F C A

S U I R A L F U A C B A M A T R B A

P L T A E V N O L T L F A C A H A P

K J A S N A L I M D R A N T U S T I

Words:

Single-task

Mindful

Slow

Self-care

Calm

Reading

Immersing yourself in the pages of a good book, whether it's a romance novel or a practical guide to archery, helps to calm the mind and slows us down. Nicholas Carr, author of *The Shallows: What the Internet Is Doing to Our Brains*, hails the benefits of "deep reading" which is when we focus on a single piece of text for an extended period, saying, "book reading 'understimulates the senses' [which] makes the activity so intellectually rewarding. By allowing us to filter out distractions, to quiet the problem-solving functions of the frontal lobes, deep reading becomes a form of deep thinking".

Books are like old friends – reliable, loyal, endlessly interesting and good for you. Cultivate your bookshelf with new and insightful books, ones that surprise you and test you, and ones that make you feel a sense of belonging, knowing that they are friends for life.

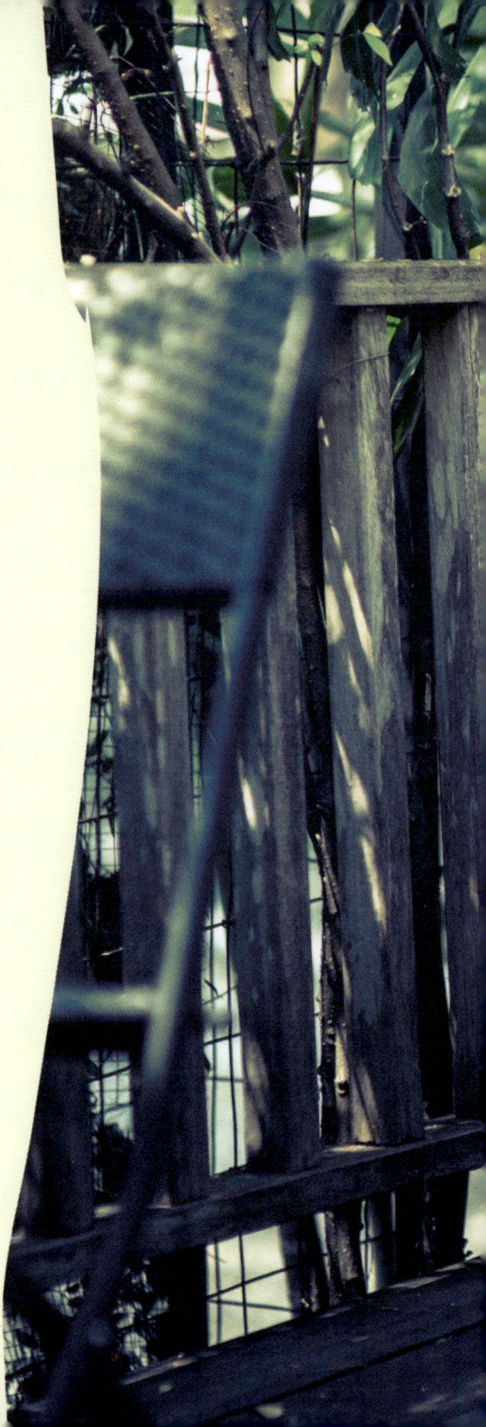

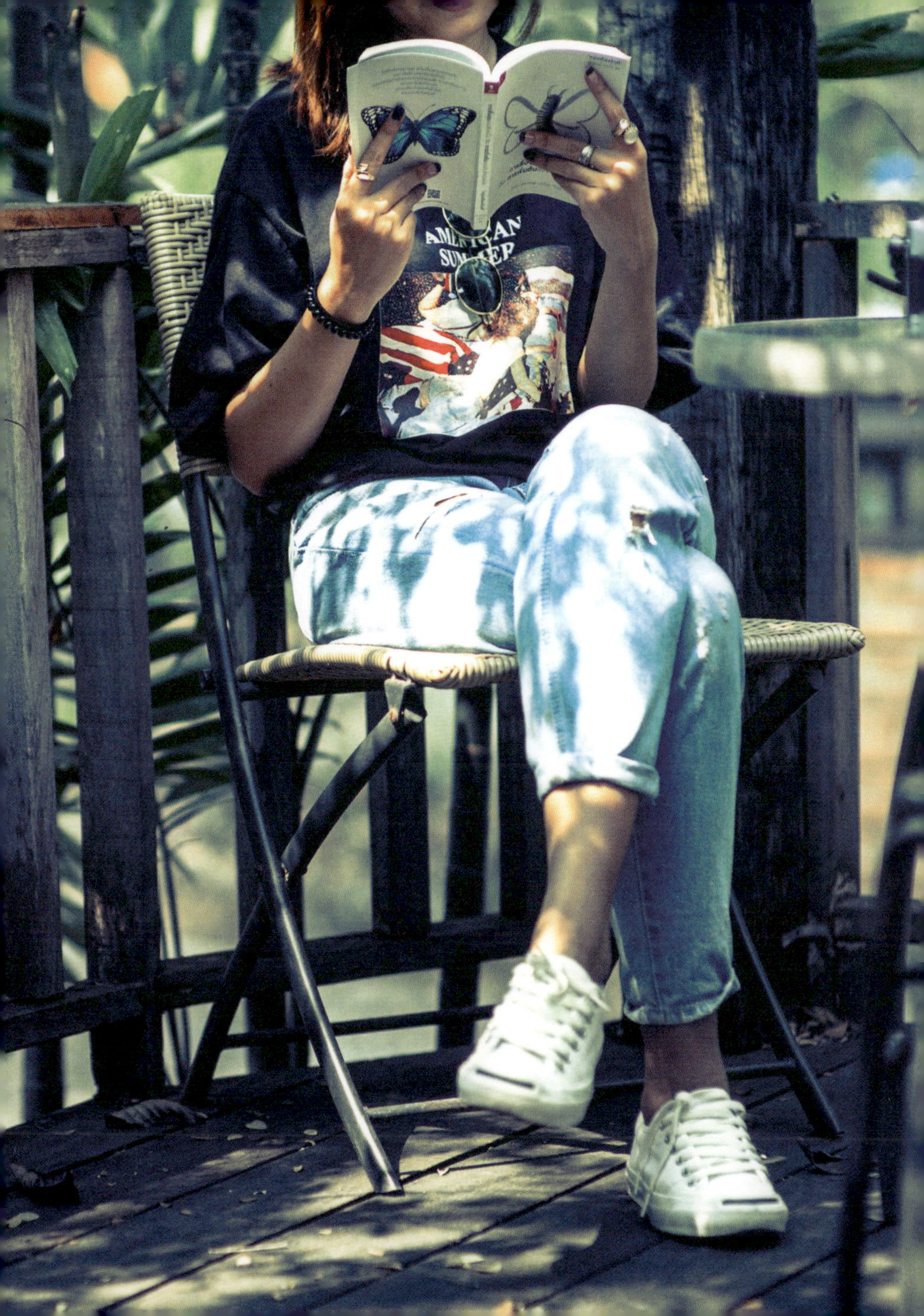

Tips for slow moments of creativity

If you normally watch TV or browse the internet of an evening, try switching off screens and devices for one or two evenings a week and instead try your hand at some creative pursuits. Here are some simple ideas to explore.

Write a five-line poem about someone you know – it could be an amusing limerick

Memorize a favourite *poem*

Print out photos from your phone and frame them, or begin a photo album

Write a letter to a friend who you haven't seen in a while

Listen to a podcast

Do some *mending* – sew on buttons, darn holes in socks, replace a zip

Read newspaper or magazine articles that you have saved and haven't got around to reading

Write a diary entry

Look at the stars and learn the constellations

Carefully *observe* an object in pencil or paint

Learn to interpret your *dreams*

Plant some seeds

Learn some phrases for an upcoming foreign holiday using language books

Read a chapter of a book

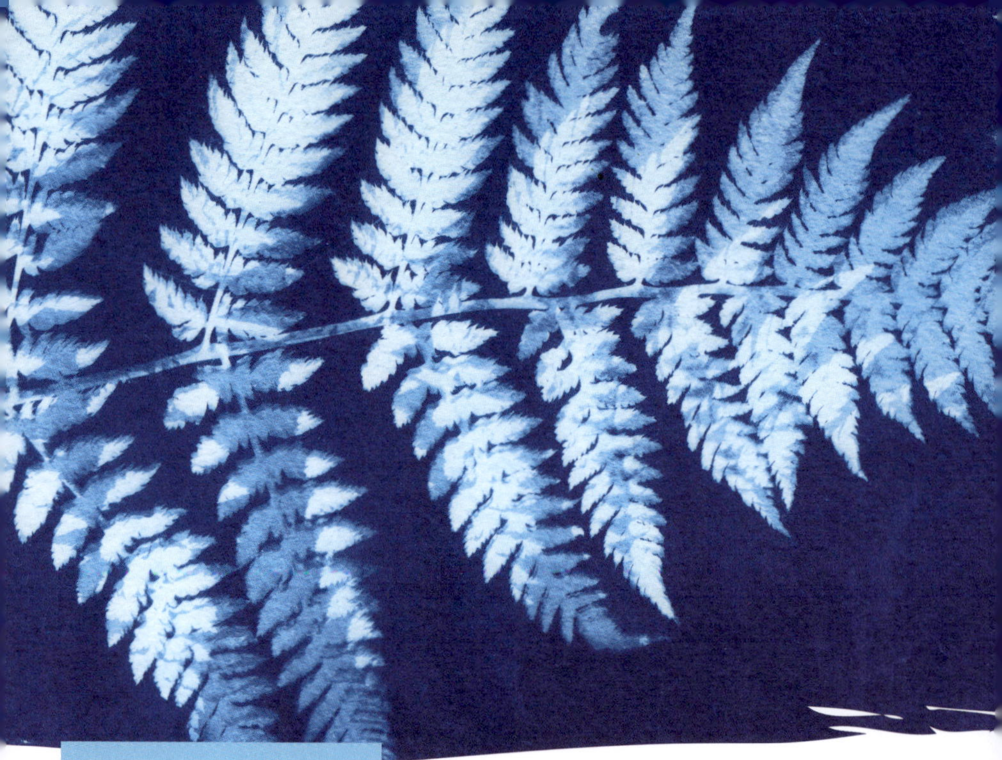

Capture a moment

Thanks to smartphones, people tend to have a camera on them most of the time. Taking photos helps you to focus on being in the present moment as you notice the little things that surround you, such as colours in the sky, birds flying, the play of light, shadows cast and funny expressions. Get in the habit of taking just a handful of photos a day so that you stop to focus and capture those fleeting moments that normally pass us by.

There are "slower" methods of taking photographs than with a phone. Try sun prints, where you place objects over a piece of prepared photo paper in the sunshine and leave for a few minutes before immersing the paper in water to create a beautiful cobalt-coloured print. And, of course, there is the old-school film camera – having a limited number of images to take encourages careful consideration before taking each shot.

SLOW MOMENT

Stop and take a moment
to admire all the beautiful
things you take for
granted every day.

SLOW EXERCISE

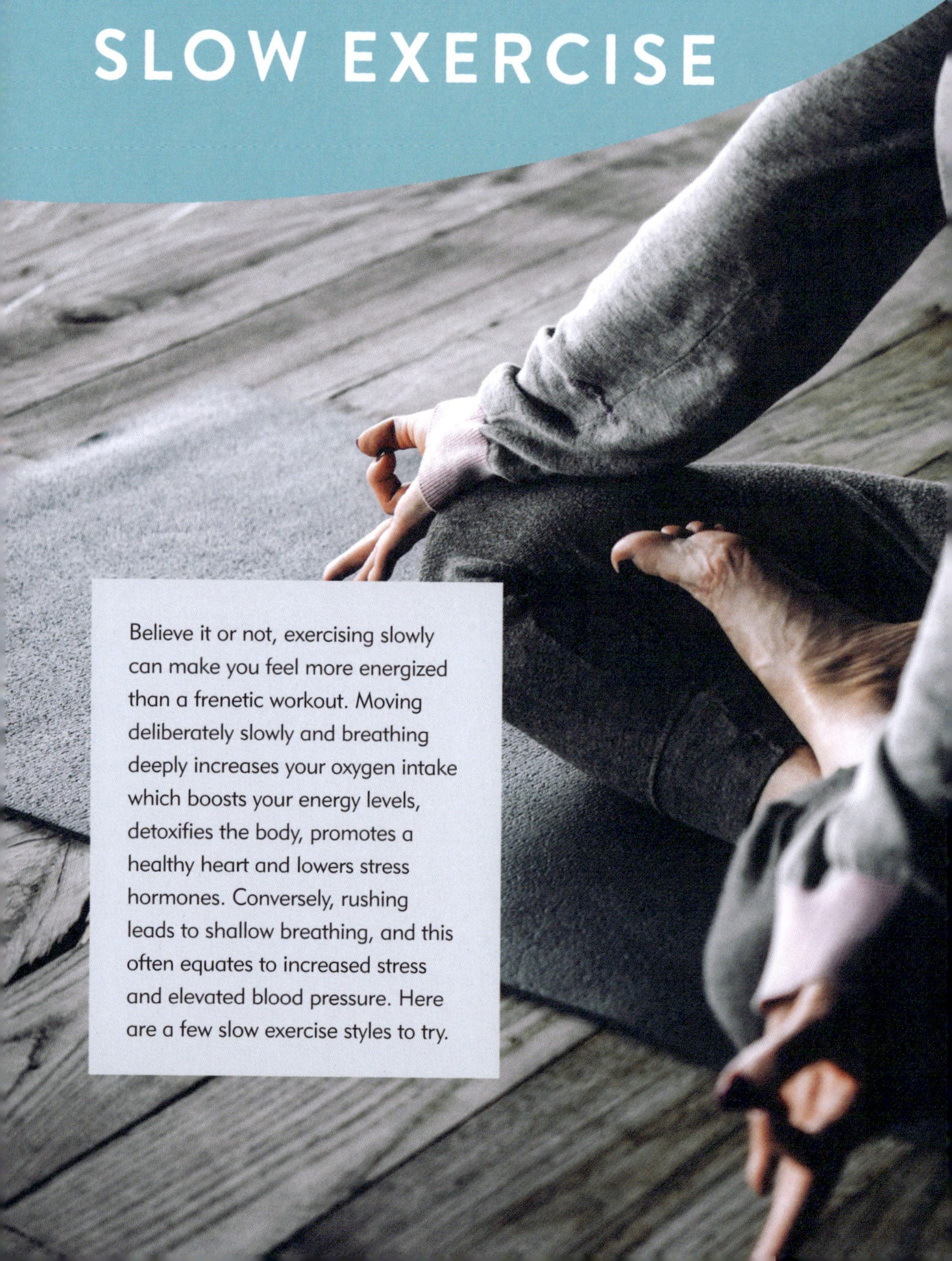

Believe it or not, exercising slowly can make you feel more energized than a frenetic workout. Moving deliberately slowly and breathing deeply increases your oxygen intake which boosts your energy levels, detoxifies the body, promotes a healthy heart and lowers stress hormones. Conversely, rushing leads to shallow breathing, and this often equates to increased stress and elevated blood pressure. Here are a few slow exercise styles to try.

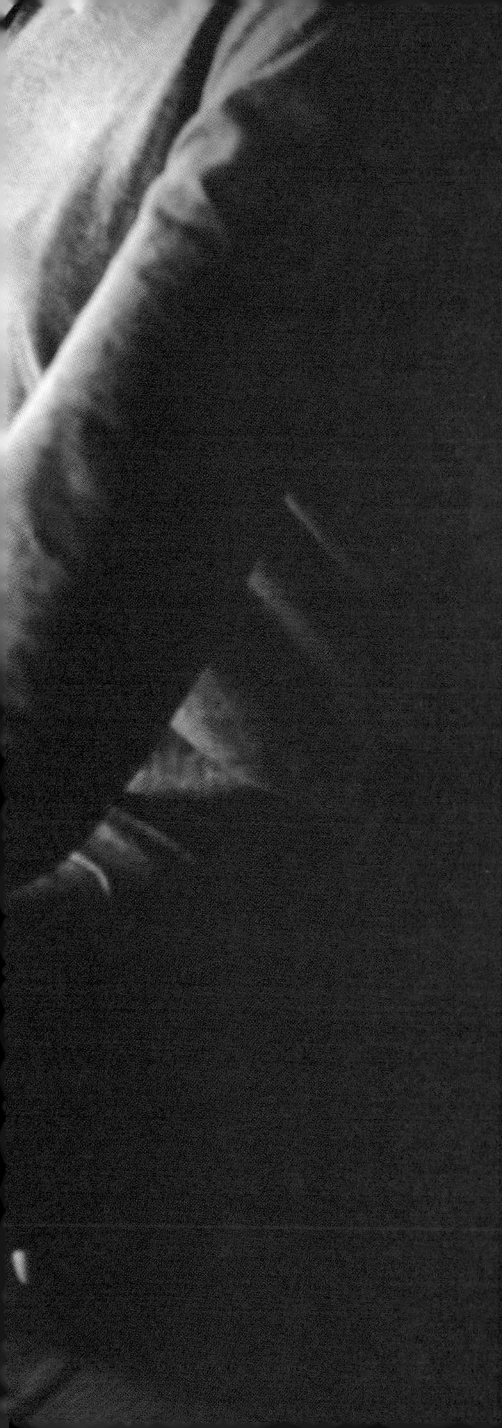

YOGA

This is the most obvious slow exercise, along with tai chi and Pilates. Performing slow, deliberate movements helps to calm the mind and strengthen your body as well as improve posture, balance and flexibility. This form of stretching has been shown to ease the symptoms of arthritis and decrease back pain and chronic pain, but before you start any new exercise, consult your doctor if you have any concerns.

Try these poses to awaken your body and mind, deepen your breathing and improve breath control. Try to do yoga in a room with natural light so that you are greeting the day. Connect each movement to an inhale or exhale of breath. These are the postures you will need to learn for a sun salutation.

Mountain Pose

TADASANA

While this may look like you're simply standing up straight, this surprisingly strong pose is an important one. It will help you to find your space on the mat, ground you to the earth and connect you back to your breath.

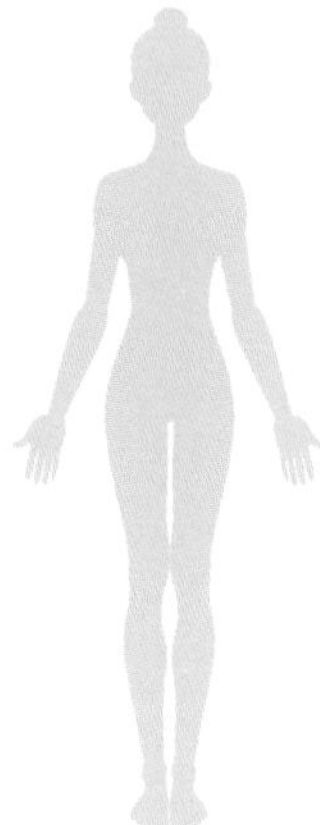

1. Stand at the top of your mat with your heels together. Place your arms down by your sides with your palms facing in. Fingers should be engaged as they lengthen towards the mat.
2. Close your eyes and take a moment to bring your attention to each area of your body. Start by lifting your toes, spreading them wide apart and then lowering them back onto the mat, becoming aware of each toe connected to the mat. Then notice the balls and soles of your feet as you spread your weight evenly over each foot.
3. Straighten your legs, ensure your knees are directly over your ankles and your hips are directly over your knees. Engage your thighs, lifting your kneecaps and strengthening your legs. Support this movement by tucking your tail bone under and engaging your core (abdominal muscles).
4. Now take your attention to your spine, feel yourself lifting and lengthening as you draw the crown of your head towards the sky. Open your chest as you roll your shoulders back, lengthening your arms at your sides.
5. Draw your chin slightly down to lengthen the back of your neck. Stand tall and connect to your breathing.

Deep Forward Fold Pose

UTTANASANA

This deep fold gives an intense stretch to your hamstrings and spine, and allows a softening in your neck and shoulders, increasing the blood flow to your brain, helping you to calm your mind and feel restored and refreshed.

1. Stand in Mountain Pose at the top of your mat. Inhale as you lift your arms above your head, joining your palms together. Allow your gaze to follow your arms as they lift, watching your palms as they join.
2. Tuck your tailbone under and engage your lower belly. Exhale as you fold forwards, hinging from the hips. Keep drawing your navel back towards your spine and make your spine long as you fold towards the knees.
3. Place your hands on the floor either side of your feet. If you can't reach your hands to the floor, bend your knees a little. Press your palms to the floor, spreading your fingers and engaging with your mat.
4. Draw your shoulders back, lengthening your neck, and tuck your chin slightly under. Allow gravity to draw the crown of your head closer to the mat.
5. Take five deep breaths. If your legs are bent, allow them to gently straighten with each exhale.
6. Inhale as you lift up again bringing your palms back together above your head. Exhale as you lower your hands to come into Mountain Pose.

Downward-Facing Dog Pose

ADHO MUKHA SVANASANA

One of the most widely recognized yoga poses, Downward-Facing Dog, is ideal for an all-over energizing stretch.

1. Come onto your mat on your hands and knees, with your knees directly below your hips and your hands slightly above your shoulders. Spread your fingers, and connect your palms and each fingertip with the mat.
2. Tuck your toes under and lift your knees away from the mat, start to lengthen and lift your tailbone away from your pelvis, lifting your sitting bones towards the ceiling.
3. Push your thighs back, feel your chest softening back towards your knees and draw your heels towards the floor. Straighten your legs but be careful not to lock your knees.
4. Draw your shoulders away from your ears, widening your shoulder blades and drawing them back towards your tail-bone. Feel your spine lengthen and straighten, keeping your back flat. Your head should be between your upper arms, with your gaze towards your navel.
5. Hold pose for five deep breaths, then bend your knees back down to the mat and draw your sitting bones back towards your heels.

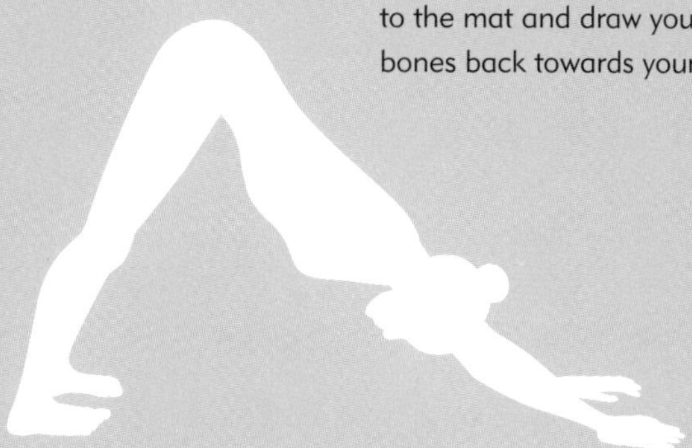

Upward-Facing Dog Pose

URDHVA MUKHA SVANASANA

Upward-Facing Dog is a rejuvenating stretch that works your whole spine, opens your chest, tones your belly and strengthens your arms and wrists.

1. Lie flat, with your forehead resting on the mat, and the tops of your feet flat to the mat and hip-width apart.
2. Place your hands to the sides of your body, palms flat to the mat, fingers pointing forwards with your fingertips in line with your shoulders. Tuck your toes under and inhale as you press your hands into the mat and lift your body away from the floor. Start to pull your hips forwards as you roll over your toes so the tops of your feet are flat to the mat again.
3. Straighten your arms and lift your chest forwards: feel like you're pulling your chest through your arms. Make sure your legs are straight and engaged, keeping the thighs and knees lifted off the mat. The weight of your body should be spread evenly over your hands and feet.
4. Roll your shoulders back and down, tilt your head back slightly and take your gaze up.
5. Soften your shoulders, pulling them down your back, opening across the chest. Tuck your chin in towards your throat, keeping the neck long.
6. Hold for five deep breaths, expanding your chest and lengthening your spine with each breath. To release, bend your knees to the mat and exhale as you slowly lower all the way down to the mat.

Four-Limbed Staff Pose

CHATURANGA DANDASANA

This pose is great for full-body strengthening. As the weight of your body rests on your hands and feet, you are working your arms, wrists, shoulders and core.

1. Start on your mat in a plank position, with your shoulders stacked above your wrists, fingers pointing forwards, feet hip distance apart. Push your heels back, ensuring your shoulders and wrists are still stacked.
2. Engage your abdominal muscles and slowly start to move the shoulders forwards to your fingertips as you bend into your elbows. Before lowering, turn your inner elbows to face into each other to keep them hugged into the body and avoid them pushing outwards.
3. Keep slowly lowering until your elbows are bent at right angles and the tops of your arms are in line with your chest. Ensure your whole body is straight, avoid lifting your buttocks and keep your neck in line with your spine, with your gaze lowered.
4. Hold for five deep breaths. Exhale as you slowly lower all the way down to the mat.

Cobra Pose

BHUJANGASANA

This pose is a wonderful stretch to open up your chest and stretch all across the front of your body. It stimulates your digestive organs, increases movement in your spine and strengthens your arms.

1. Lie flat, with your forehead resting onto the mat, the tops of the feet flat to the mat and your feet together.
2. Place your hands underneath your shoulders, palms flat to the mat, fingers pointing forwards. Roll your chest up and away from the mat and feel your body lengthening from the base of your belly to your chest. Engage your thigh muscles and feel your knees lifting.
3. Start to press your pubic bone down and inhale as you lift your chest higher. Keep the tops of your feet pressing down and press your palms down as you straighten your arms, curling your spine up and raising your chest. Feel the arching movement from the base of the spine to the middle of your back. Plant the heels of your hands into the mat so you feel almost like you are pulling your chest forwards.
4. Soften your shoulders, pulling them down your back, opening across the chest. Tuck your chin in towards your throat, keeping the neck long. Hold for five deep breaths, expanding your chest and lengthening your spine with each breath. Exhale as you slowly lower all the way down to the mat.

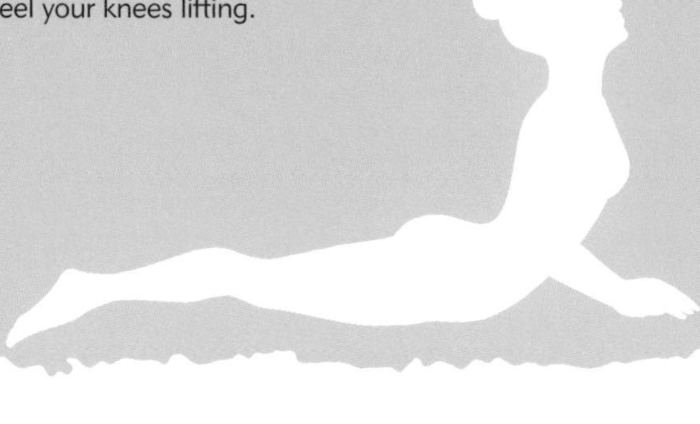

Breathe in calm with affirmations

Whether you're in your comfiest chair at home or about to give a presentation at the office, you can introduce a slow moment with a breathing meditation to bring a sense of calm wherever you are.

Start by becoming aware of your breath as it enters and leaves your nostrils. Breathe to your own rhythm. After a few breaths, focus on breathing in and breathing out the feelings you wish to nurture:

I breathe in calm. I breathe out calm.

I breathe in peace. I breathe out peace.

I breathe in love. I breathe out love.

I breathe in strength. I breathe out strength.

I breathe in harmony. I breathe out harmony.

Create as many lines to your meditation as you wish, using words that are meaningful to you and the situation you find yourself in. This meditation is especially helpful if you're about to do something you feel nervous about: a job interview, a meeting with your child's teacher or any other important task.

Everything you
do can be done

better

from a place of

relaxation.

STEPHEN C. PAUL

SWIMMING

Swimming is one of the most effective forms of exercise, both in terms of giving you a full-body workout and in allowing you to relax and slow down. The rhythmic lap of the water with each stroke, and the focus on your technique and breathing, really make this a great way to move your mind away from your worries and to allow some quality time to yourself. Swimming can be enjoyed slowly while still reaping the benefits for health and well-being. A study made by Indiana University demonstrated that those in middle age and beyond who swim regularly are biologically 20 years younger than their birth age, as this exercise lowers blood pressure and cholesterol levels, and improves agility, flexibility and brain function.

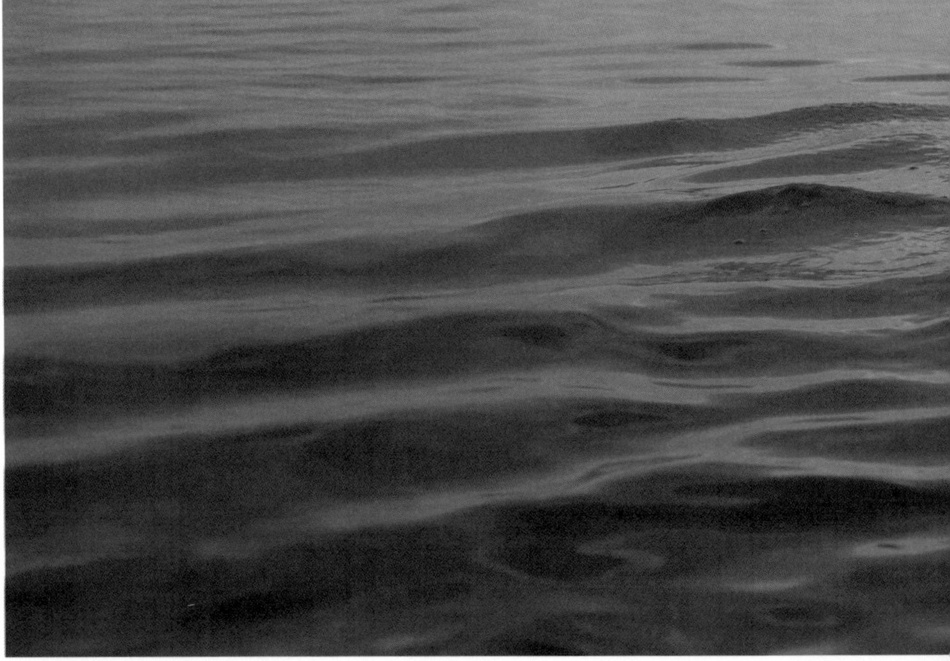

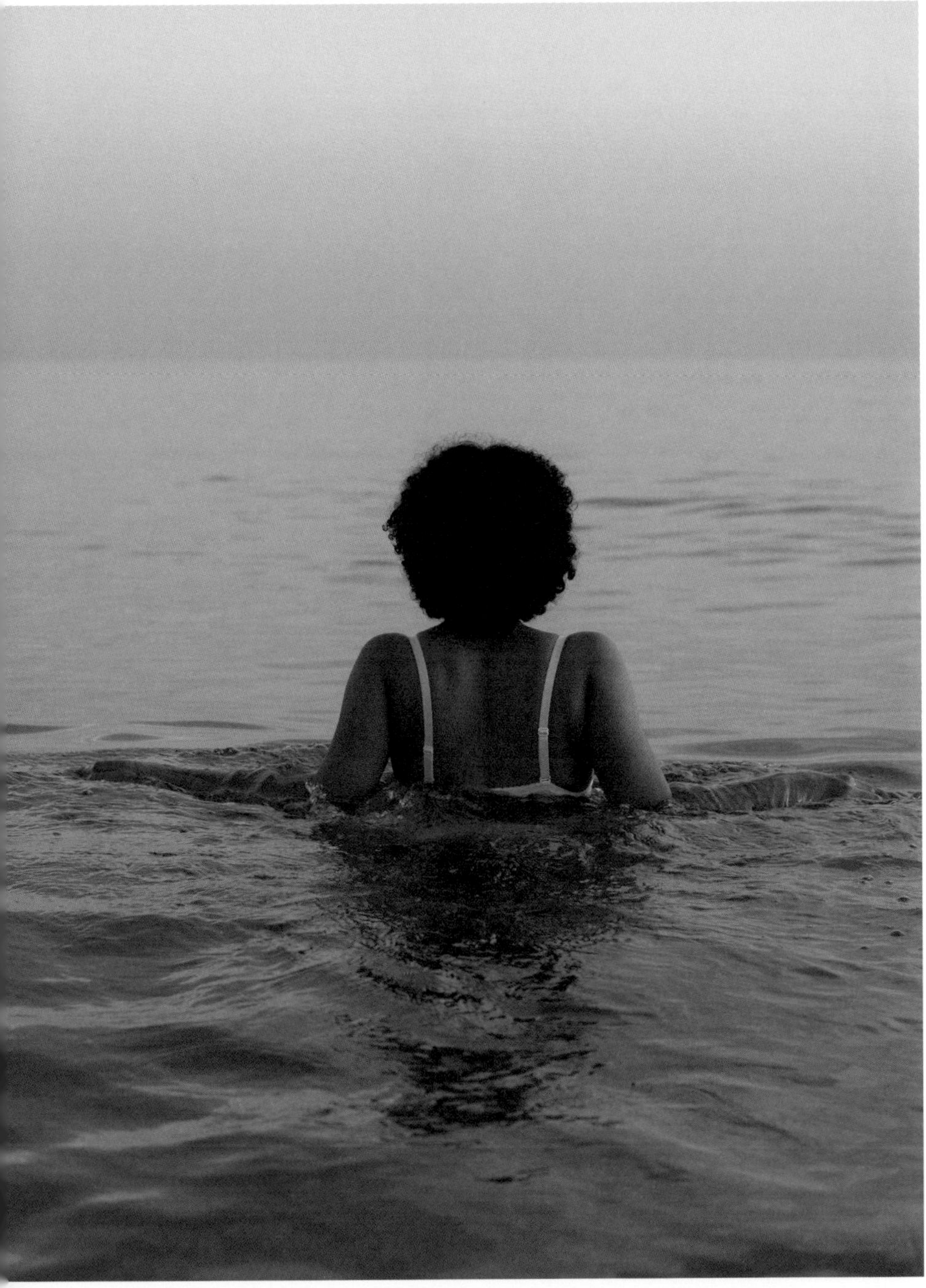

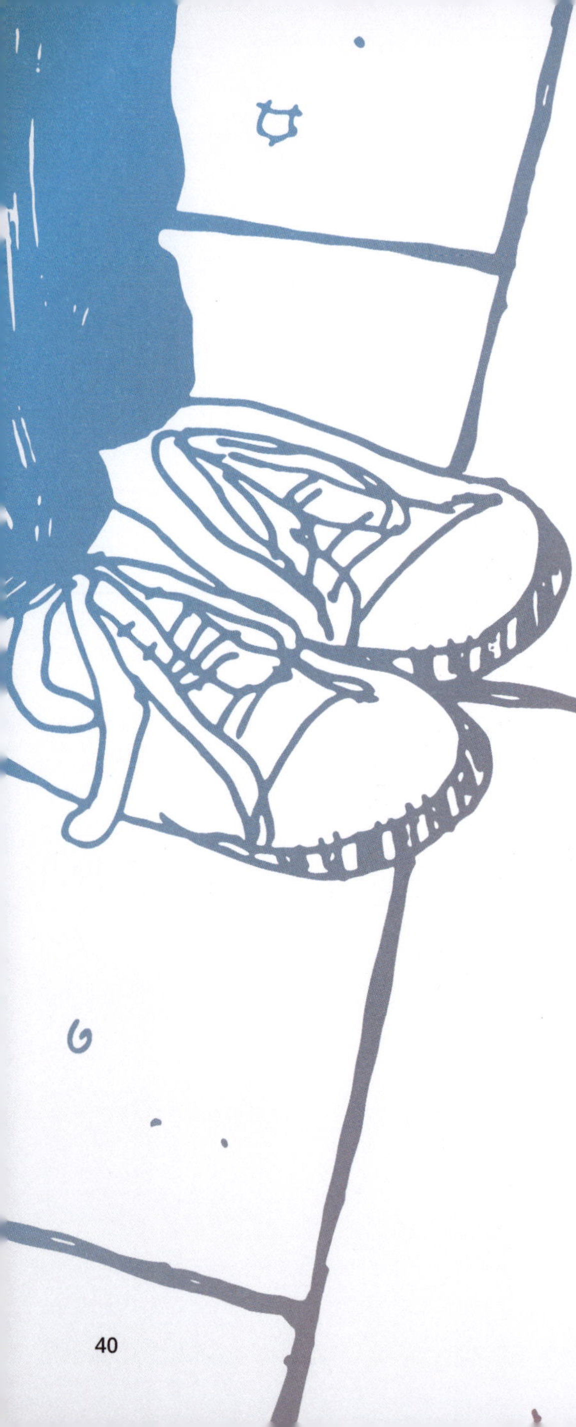

Walking

Soak up the great outdoors and go out for a walk. This is one of the best ways to appreciate living slowly. Walking with no particular purpose and without time constraints can be the ultimate way to de-stress, whether it's ambling through the side streets of your local town or hiking up hills and stopping every so often to admire the view and listen to the birds or the wind in the trees. Walking is restorative, therapeutic and rewarding in so many ways. Experts from Saarland University in Germany reported to the European Society of Cardiology Congress in 2015 that just 25 minutes of walking a day can add up to seven years to your life.

Birdsong

Birds are everywhere, but how often do you stop to notice and appreciate them? Birdwatching is another cue to help slow your pace. Pay close attention to the sound of birdsong accompanying you as you go about your day.

SLOW MOMENT

Close your eyes and listen for 1 minute to all the sounds around you. For 1 minute, you have nothing else to do but listen.

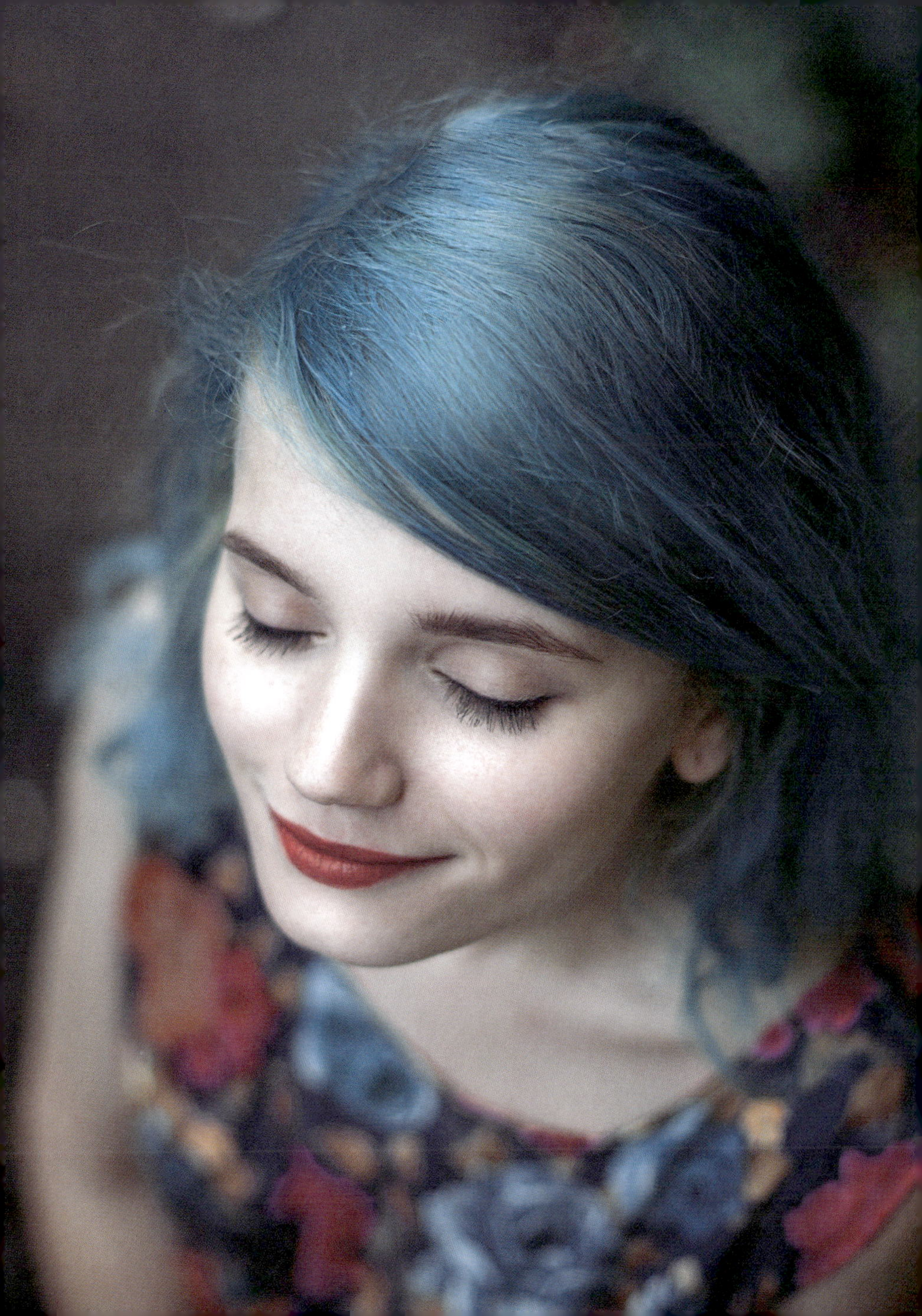

SELF-CARE

Self-care is intrinsic to living slowly, as the values and aims of both are the same: to protect or nurture your own health and well-being. Taking the time for self-care in your day-to-day life is a big step towards a happy, healthy and stress-free life. Acts of self-care can be anything from completing mundane everyday tasks – like having a daily beauty regime and doing the washing up – to making sure you take time out to rest and feel good – such as indulging in a long bath, calling a friend for a chat, or taking your whole lunch break to go for a walk or read a book instead of spending it at your desk. The small things are just as important as the bigger things in keeping you balanced and feeling well, and it's at the times when you feel most pressured that you need to remember this the most. Practising self-care is vital to achieve the bigger goals, because you need to focus on yourself first in order to progress in life. Begin gently with these ideas.

DO A BODY SWEEP

Research shows that our emotions manifest in our body. For example, negative emotions often cause people to tense the muscles in their jaw and around their eyes and mouth. With repeated stress, these muscles can become sore and tight. One of the key ways to balance your mind–body connection is to stop and give yourself a "body sweep". Sit quietly and systematically scan your body, starting at the top of your head and moving down over your face, the back of your neck, your shoulders, arms, hands, torso, hips, legs and feet. As you do this, notice the sensations you feel. Are there any areas of tension, pressure or discomfort? If so, breathe into these areas and allow them to soften and relax. Practising this body sweep on a regular basis can help you become more alert to the messages of your body. The tension you discover might be a "gut feeling" about a choice you're making or a headache may indicate that you need to pay attention to a health issue. By exploring the link between your body and mind, you will start to notice which parts of the body are stimulated or shut down when you experience a particular emotion. "Softening" these areas can help release the tension or emotion stored there.

HOW ARE YOU FEELING?

It's a simple question, and it's one that we often ask others but not ourselves. Make a point of asking yourself once or twice a day – so you are checking in with how you are feeling. If the answer to the question is on the spectrum of "I've been better", don't ignore it – do something about it, so that you feel good. Equally, listen to your body – if you sense you need a rest or some time to de-stress, don't ignore these important cues.

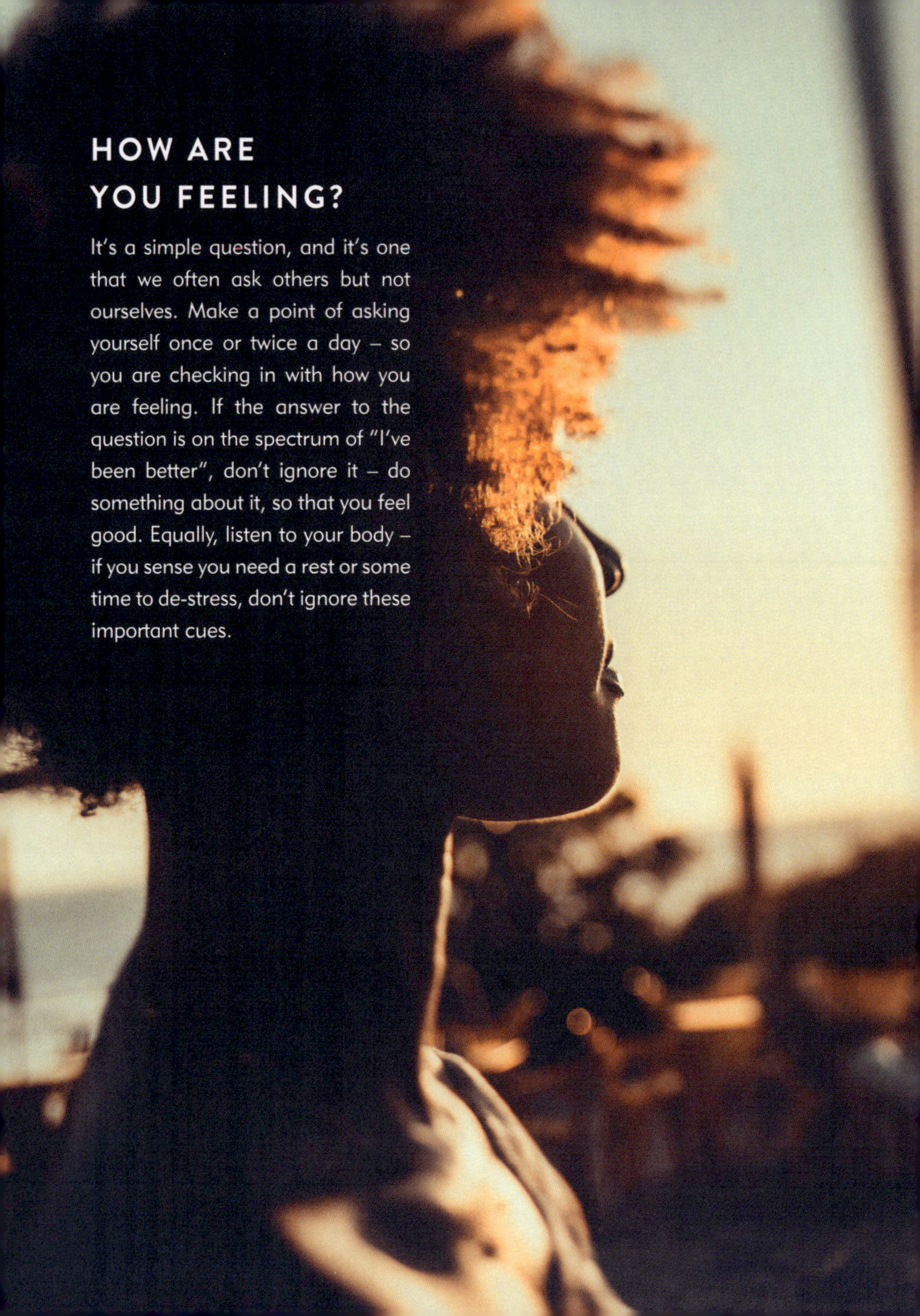

GET ENOUGH SLEEP

This isn't always possible, but try to set up the best conditions to ensure you get a good night's sleep. Most adults need between 7 and 9 hours a night, but everyone is different. The best way to ascertain how much sleep you need is to listen to your body. Regardless of whether you're meeting the recommended guidelines or not, if you feel rested, you're probably getting enough sleep, and if you are tired and sluggish, you're probably not.

Tips to help you sleep well:

- Write down your worries before you go to sleep so they're not replaying in your mind and keeping you awake.
- Plan as much as you can for the next day before you go to bed – this could include preparing breakfast, deciding what to wear and writing a to-do list.
- Make your bedroom a healthy and enticing sanctuary with bed linen that feels nice on your skin, and pillows and a mattress that give the right support. Decorate in calm, neutral tones rather than ones that will stimulate the senses.
- Keep your bedroom a screen- and gadget-free zone, and aim to switch off your gadgets at least half an hour before going to bed.

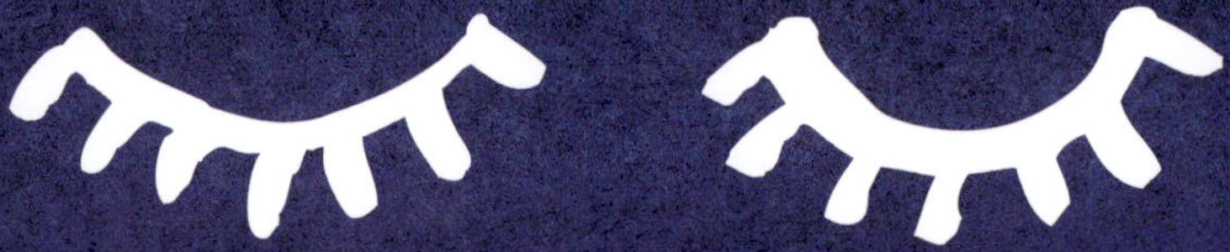

NO MORE JUNK SLEEP

The term "junk sleep" was coined by researchers in Singapore to refer to the inability to achieve REM sleep due to excessive screen time before going to bed. We know from numerous studies that this is bad for us, but around 78 per cent of adults check their phones within the hour before going to bed. The blue light from screens can disrupt melatonin production and increase cortisol that keeps us awake causing disturbed sleep, which increases the risk of poor mental health, memory loss and depression. The brain needs a minimum of 5 hours of sleep a night to clean up toxins that have accumulated throughout the day. It has also been suggested in a study carried out by the National Institute of Environmental Health Sciences in the USA that it's important to keep your phone a few feet away from your bed to avoid unnecessary low-level radiation, which can affect the function of the nervous system. Research from Brigham and Women's Hospital in Massachusetts concluded that reading from a screen before going to sleep has a significant impact on how alert you are the following day.

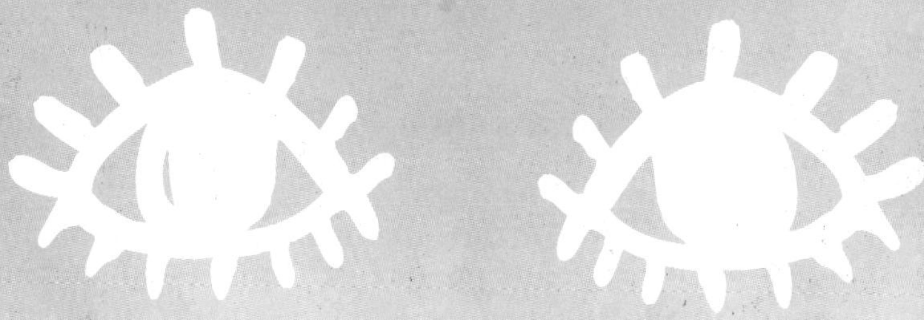

GET UP EARLIER

No, not so you can get more work done – an earlier start will make the morning routine less rushed and maybe even enjoyable and something to look forward to. Be kind to your future self and plan a nutritious breakfast the night before, maybe even making it the night before too – such as overnight oats (see page 98). Use the extra time to sit in your favourite spot and enjoy your breakfast rather than grabbing something on the go. Having a little more time in the morning could also give you the opportunity to create a more inspirational lunch, such as a healthy superfood salad (see page 109).

SLOW MOMENT

As you get dressed and undressed, slow down and notice the textures of the fabric and how they feel on your skin. Use calm, unhurried movements.

Take a deep breath. Get present in the moment and ask yourself what is important this very second.

GREG McKEOWN

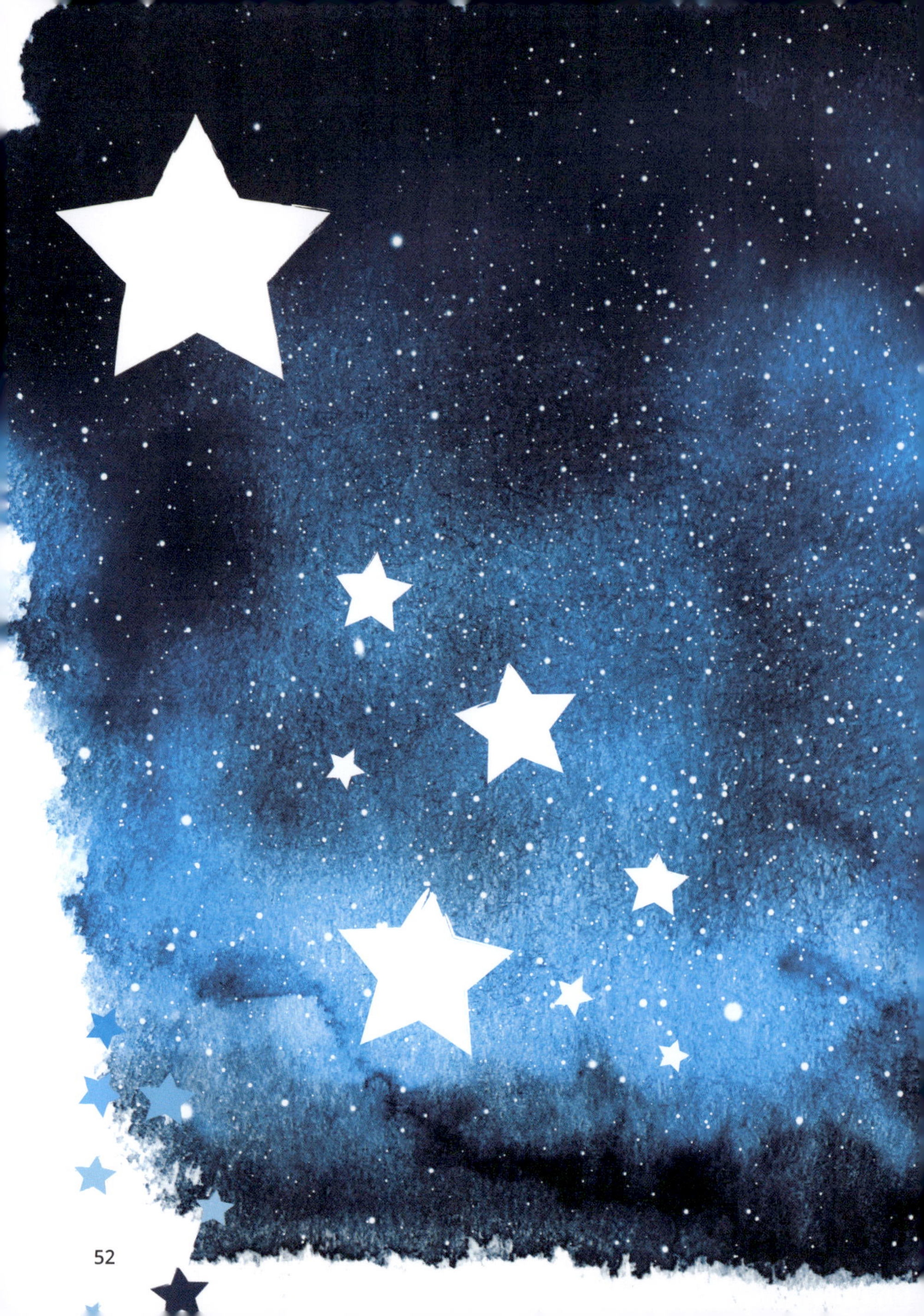

LOOK UP

If you feel like the walls are caving in and life is too hectic to even consider slowing down, try this exercise to alter your mindset, which is part of a Buddhist teaching called "cosmic perspective". Pick an evening with a clear sky so that the stars are bright. Go to a quiet place with minimal light pollution, such as a beach or a hillside away from a town, and sit peacefully while gazing at the sky. Try to clear your mind and lose yourself in the vastness of the heavens. Consider how you're sitting on a tiny speck called Earth, which is bobbing around in this vast black universe. Now guide your eyes down and notice life around you – there could be people walking their dogs or jogging past you – and be aware that each person carries their own problems and they may even be thinking about them as you observe them. Reflect on your own life in its entirety and feel your problems reduce in size. Gaze up again at the universe and remember how you are just a tiny part of it, and your problems carry even less weight.

TREAT YOURSELF WITH KINDNESS

Make a new habit to appreciate yourself. Take a few minutes each day to sit down with a notebook and pen and write three things in it that you feel you have done well. It can be small things like picking out an outfit for the day that really works, or cleaning something that you've been putting off, or starting a new book. With this simple activity, you'll learn to appreciate the small daily achievements as well as the big milestone moments.

> Three things in human life are important: the first is to be kind; the second is to be kind; and the third is to be kind.
>
> HENRY JAMES

TAKE YOURSELF ON A DATE

Activities like going to see a show, walking without a map, going for a morning coffee, visiting an art gallery or learning a new language all reconnect us with our creativity and passions. And if we are happier, the people around us will be happier too.

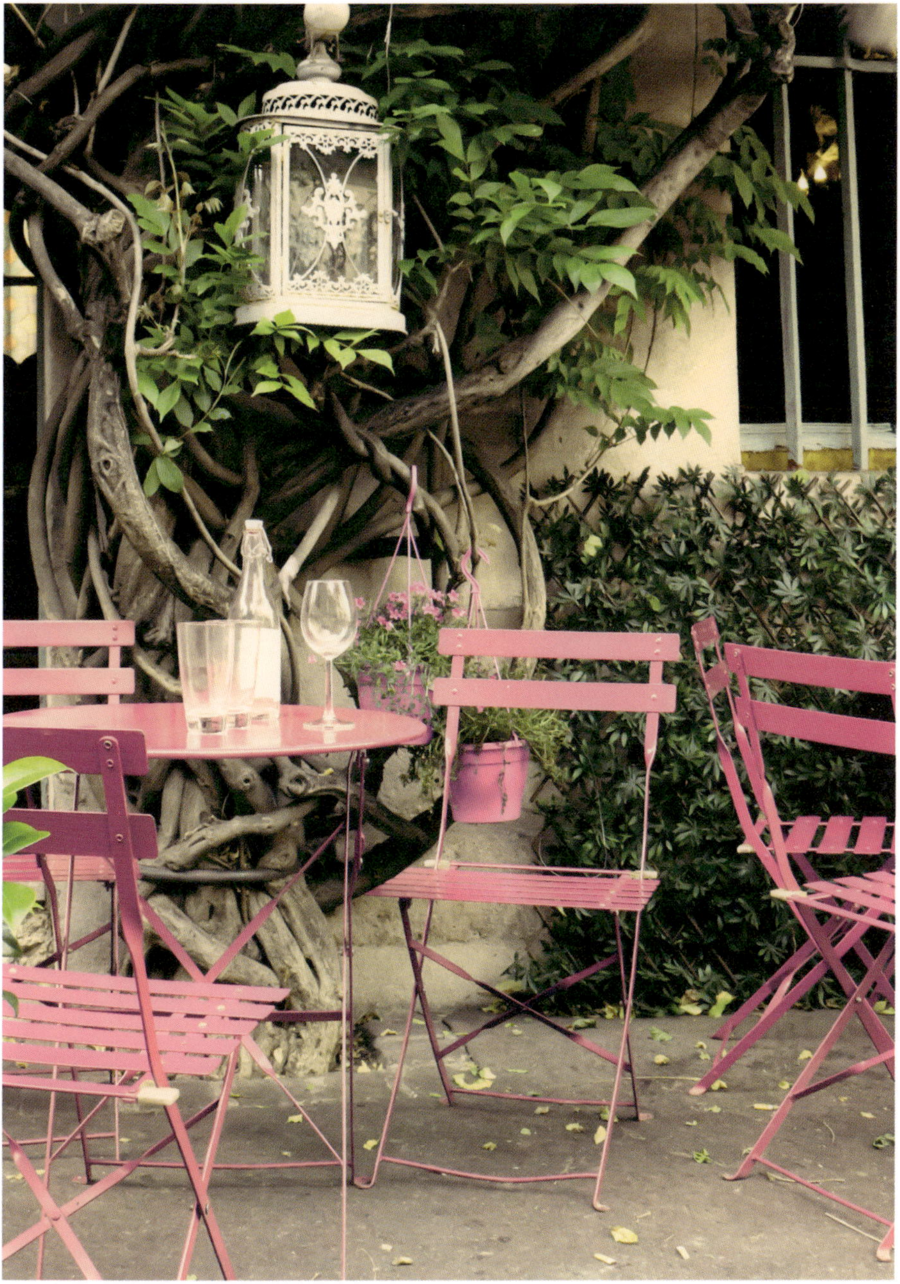

APPRECIATE NOW

Slow living encourages an appreciation for a simpler life and living in the here and now. We all experience pangs of jealousy or yearnings for what we currently don't have or can't afford, or haven't yet mastered or achieved. But if you're constantly striving for the next thing and not appreciating what you have, you'll never be happy no matter how successful you are. Making the most of what you have, and relishing and treasuring those things, is intrinsic to a happy life. Comparing yourself to others will also steer you away from looking at all the good things in your life. Emulating others will not make you happy – instead, focus on being the best version of you. Remember: the more you think you need to be happy, the harder it is to become so.

COLLECT EVERYDAY MOMENTS

It's easy to forget yourself and your needs on a day-to-day basis, but slow living encourages a more considered approach to help you define what is important to you and to think more about your well-being. Keep a scrapbook or notebook (it could be a physical book or a virtual one, such as Pinterest) and store up images, quotes and memes that truly resonate with you, or who you want to be. Make regular additions – snap a picture of a perfect sunrise on your early-morning commute, record something that made you laugh on the radio, save a tweet from a favourite author – so that you can return to these moments whenever you're in need of a spark of joy.

SAVOUR SPECIAL TIMES

Just like collecting everyday moments, recognize when something is really good, such as catching up with a good friend, going for a walk on an empty beach or watching the sun rise. Be present; soak up every detail – the colours, the sounds and meaningful words spoken.

Who am I again?

Growing up does not have to go hand in hand with becoming boring or being sensible. You may do some things differently over time – perhaps you used to be a fixture at all the party hotspots or had an unusual hobby when you were younger which might make you cringe now, but this patchwork of events and quirks are what makes you "you". Sometimes we can almost feel like we're not the same person as we used to be, and in those instances, it's time for a bit of emotional self-care. Reset your mind and do something that the "old you" really enjoyed – it could be roller-skating round the park or taking part in a rugby match – who's to say you won't experience the same euphoria the second time around?

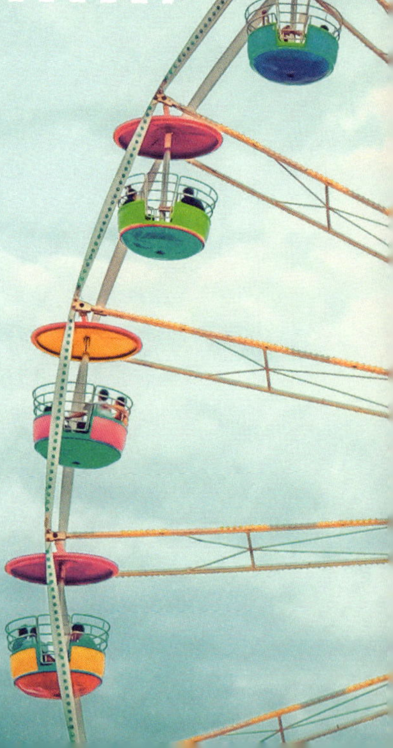

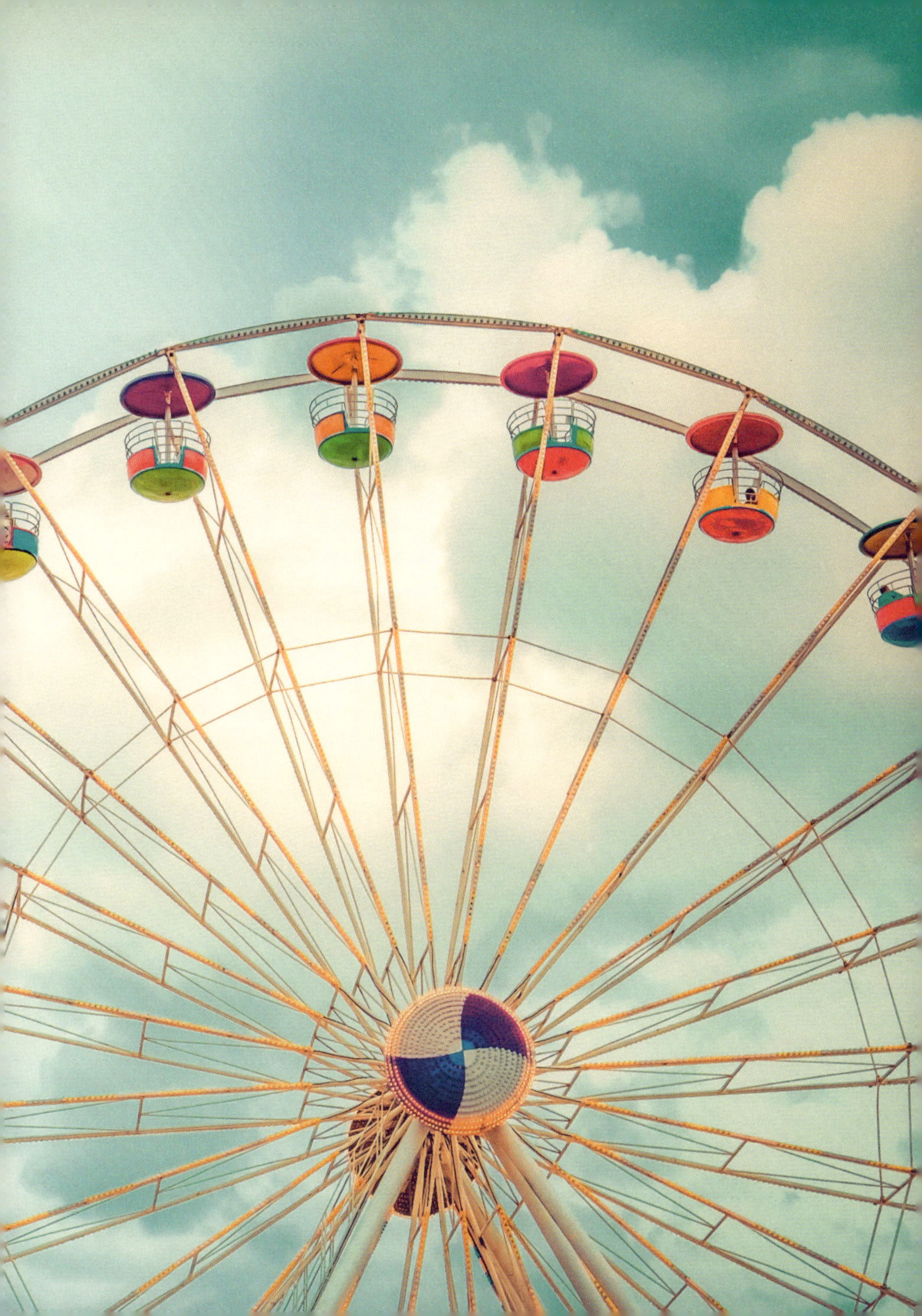

TIPS FOR A SELF-CARE STAYCATION

1 Watch some slow cinema. These are single-take films, such as a fire burning in a hearth or a railway journey

2 Hibernate for an afternoon. Put on your cosiest pyjamas and slippers

5 Enjoy silence

6 Make a self-care kit with travel-size beauty products and treats for future self-care emergencies

9 Listen to your thoughts

10 Sketch the dream you had last night

11 Stretch out on the floor

16 Plan your next holiday

17 Make yourself some tea

18 Write a diary entry

3 Enjoy a therapeutic bath with essential oils

4 Start a new book that you've been saving for a quiet moment

7 Moisturize

8 Allow yourself to sit and do nothing

12 Paint your nails

13 Clean and declutter your handbag

14 Knit a beanie

15 Make a self-care playlist of soothing music

19 Play dress-up

20 Practise yoga

21 Explore your playful side for a few moments every day and do something just for the fun of it. It could be doodling, splashing in puddles, kicking up leaves – let your imagination loose

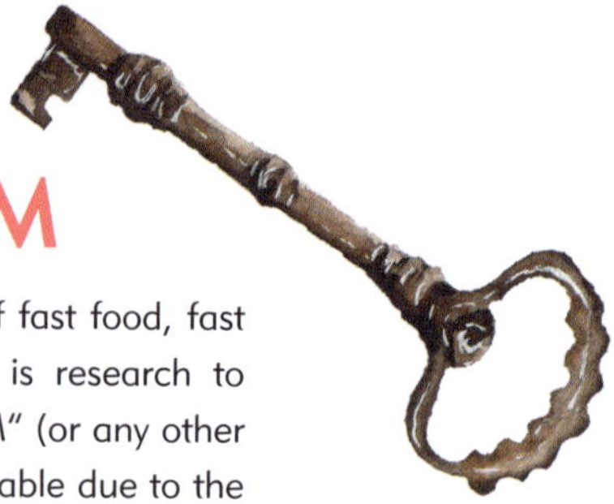

PRACTISE CALM

Impatience is the new epidemic in these times of fast food, fast fashion and high-speed internet access. There is research to suggest that even catching sight of the golden "M" (or any other fast food sign) makes a person impatient and irritable due to the habits formed by using these outlets – making quick decisions, queuing with other impatient people and eating on the hop rather than at a slow enough pace to actually enjoy it (see page 90). Consider your daily habits and how they influence your mood. Here are some ideas to introduce calm and purpose into your life by developing positive habits.

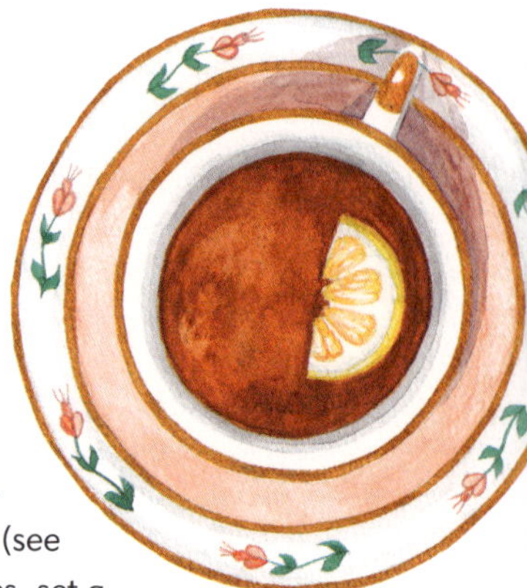

Banish the vampire time-suckers

Just as important as keeping your phone out of the bedroom – recognize when you are spending too much time in front of a screen. Stem the non-stop invasion of technology, try a digital detox and live in the moment – the world will not end if you don't check your social media feeds. Try some slow hobbies instead and nourish your mind by learning a new skill (see page 16). If you can't live without checking for updates, set a time limit on your internet usage and be strict about it.

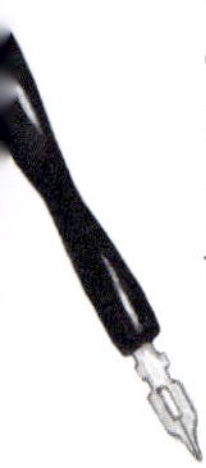

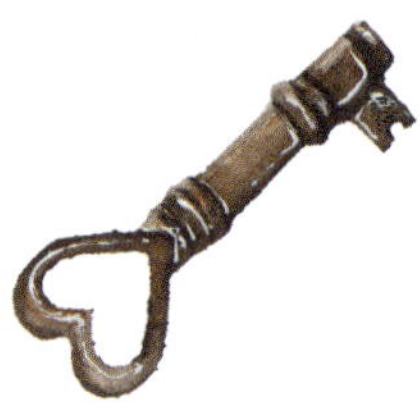

Enjoy quality time with friends

Good friendships are key to a fulfilling life. The best way to wind down and enjoy the slow lane is to spend time every day with friends and loved ones, sharing your ideas and hopes, successes and failures. Adopt mini-rituals such as arranging to meet on the same day for lunch each month, going for a run together on a Sunday morning, or simply schedule in a phone call at the same time each week.

Anything is possible when you have the right people there to support you.

MISTY COPELAND

BAD DAY?

Everyone has them.

The next time you have the day from hell, instead of wallowing in a bad mood take a simple, considered step towards bringing new ideas and fresh hopes into your life. It could be something like making a phone call or an email enquiry about a job that you're interested in, or finding a book on an area that you want to learn more about, or taking the first steps to starting a new hobby.

Slow moment

Be open to new experiences. Bring your full attention to the present moment, savouring the sights, smells and sounds of where you are.

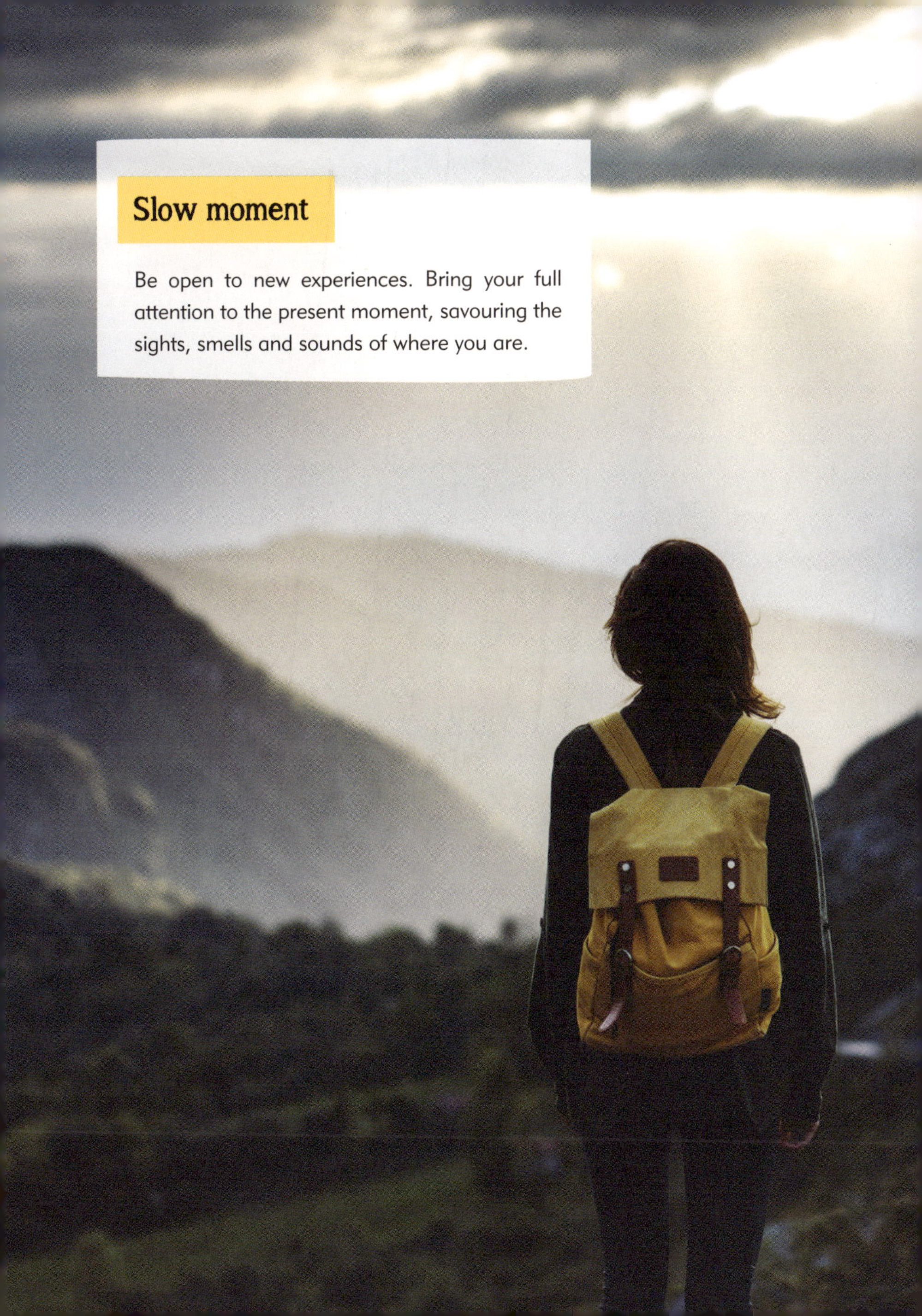

SLOW HOME

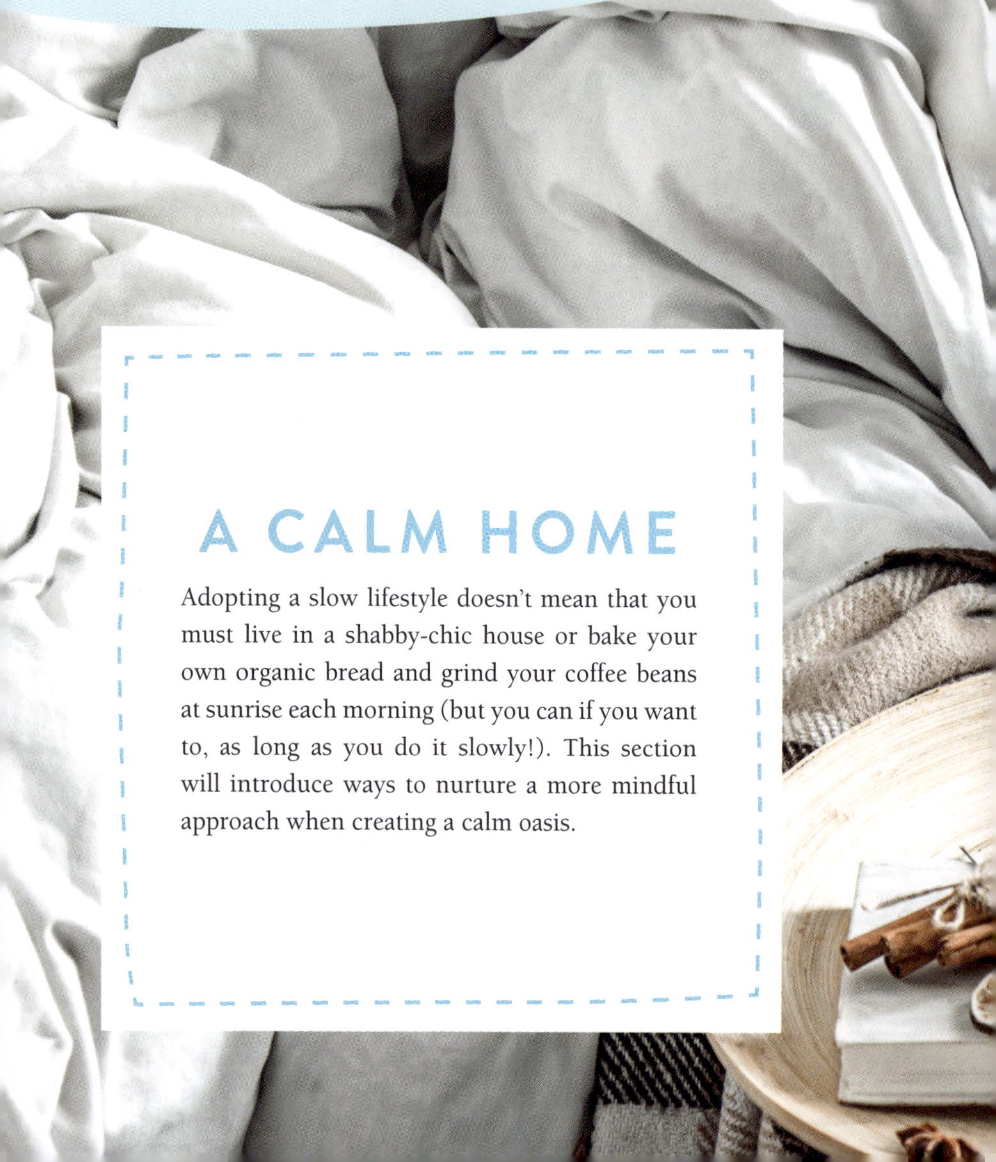

A CALM HOME

Adopting a slow lifestyle doesn't mean that you must live in a shabby-chic house or bake your own organic bread and grind your coffee beans at sunrise each morning (but you can if you want to, as long as you do it slowly!). This section will introduce ways to nurture a more mindful approach when creating a calm oasis.

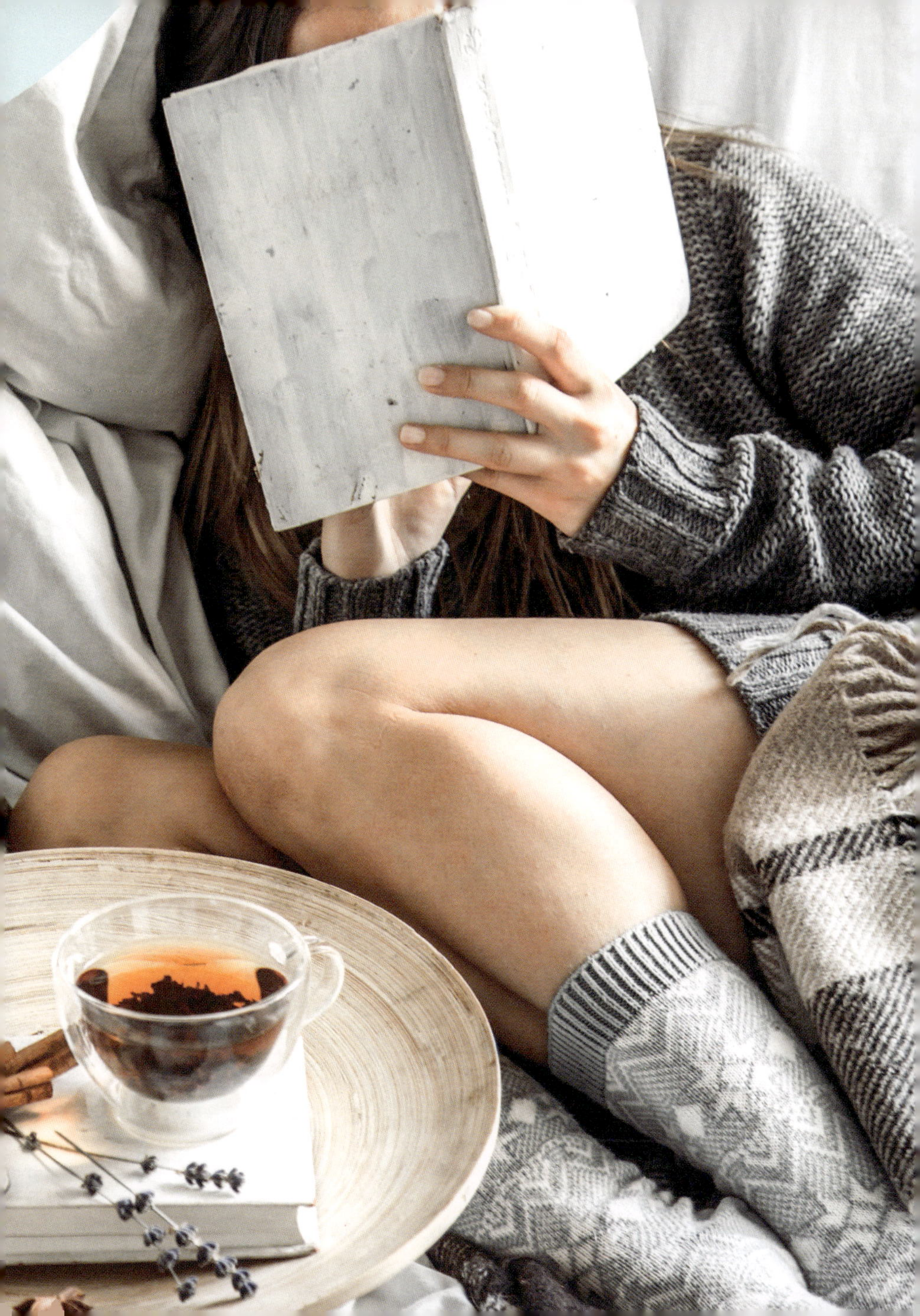

SENSE YOUR HOME

Create a slow home that harmonizes with you on all levels by focusing on the five senses. Living mindfully means engaging fully in your surroundings so it's important that you enjoy all sensations in the home. We naturally place a lot of emphasis on sight, as it's one of the senses we rely most heavily upon, but all five senses must be engaged in order to feel fully at peace in your home.

SOUND

What is the soundtrack to your home? Reconsider habits such as turning on the TV for a bit of background noise or try switching off the shuffle function on your digital music collection. Instead, put on an album and enjoy it from start to finish, whether it plays in the background as you relax after work, or you listen to it mindfully. An album is curated to evoke a mood, and is less distracting and more satisfying than throwaway TV or oft-repeated favourite tracks. Research shows that classical music in particular can help create a soothing atmosphere, as it reduces the body's production of the stress hormone cortisol. However, listening to any music that you love can help reduce anxiety and even increase brain productivity, so the most important thing is that your home is full of music that makes you happy.

TOUCH

Consider the materials you surround yourself with, especially the ones you interact with on a daily basis. Your dining table, your sofa, your sheets – they should all be made of natural materials as your body takes great pleasure from interacting with these textures. Try cotton, wool, felt and linen for your soft furnishings, blankets and sheets. Unvarnished wood is preferable for your dining table and consider using slate or cork for your coasters. Materials such as wood and cork are durable. A solid wood dining table may cost a little more but it will last a long time and take a lot of wear; an essential quality for furniture at the heart of your slow household. Natural materials are more eco-friendly too as they use fewer of the processes that involve environmentally harmful chemicals and carbon emissions.

TASTE

Fill your table with fresh food. Don't overbuy for the fruit bowl and the vegetable drawer because unused food will go to waste. Pick up seasonal fruit and vegetables every few days from local markets and vendors according to your needs. Grow a few of your own herb varieties; most herb plants don't need much space and many plants can be grown indoors. Try chives, parsley, sage, mint or oregano. Sit them on a south-facing windowsill so they get plenty of sun (a minimum of 4 hours a day) and ensure they have enough drainage by keeping the pots on a saucer. Being able to readily access fresh herbs will cut the cost of your weekly shops, improve the flavour of your meals and may even inspire you on the perennial puzzle of what to cook for dinner tonight.

SMELL

A well lived-in home will likely be subject to a jumble of smells, with the pleasant scents of a productive kitchen clashing with the less enjoyable necessities such as cleaning products or artificially scented air fresheners. Try to avoid these synthetic smells where you can and instead air your home where possible; open windows when the temperature allows (even a gust of fresh winter air can benefit a toasty but stale room) and swap the aerosols for oil-diffusing sticks. Scientists are turning their attention to household cleaning agents, with a US study identifying them as sources of urban air pollution. These chemical cleaning products and perfumes contain something called "volatile organic compounds"; when these VOCs hit the air they react with other chemicals and the result can create a whole raft of potential issues. Some people experience breathing problems due to restricted airways and there is evidence to show that the resulting particles could contribute to heart and lung disease. Be kind to your body by using natural alternatives when cleaning, such as vinegar and baking soda. Plant rosemary, lavender and lemon balm outside your front door; these fragrant herbs will gently perfume the air all year round.

SIGHT

Your surroundings should be visually pleasing and as suited to your taste as possible. However, you don't have to be perfectly on-trend in order to create a home that you're happy to look at. One long-term workplace study showed that when people work in conditions that suit their personality they experience a positive mood and improved well-being. This is important in the workplace and even more crucial in your home, which should be a nurturing haven. Your home should be an extension of your personality; if colour makes your heart leap then fill the house with colour and if you prefer cool monochromes then play with that in your interior designs. Prioritize happy memories and positive emotions in your design plans and include at least one item of emotional significance in every room of your home. This could be a book of recipes handed down through the generations and placed on a shelf in the kitchen, a well-loved blanket draped over the arm of your sofa or some driftwood taken from a coastal walk incorporated into the knick-knacks on your dresser. Every room will sing with happy memories, completing the harmony of your home.

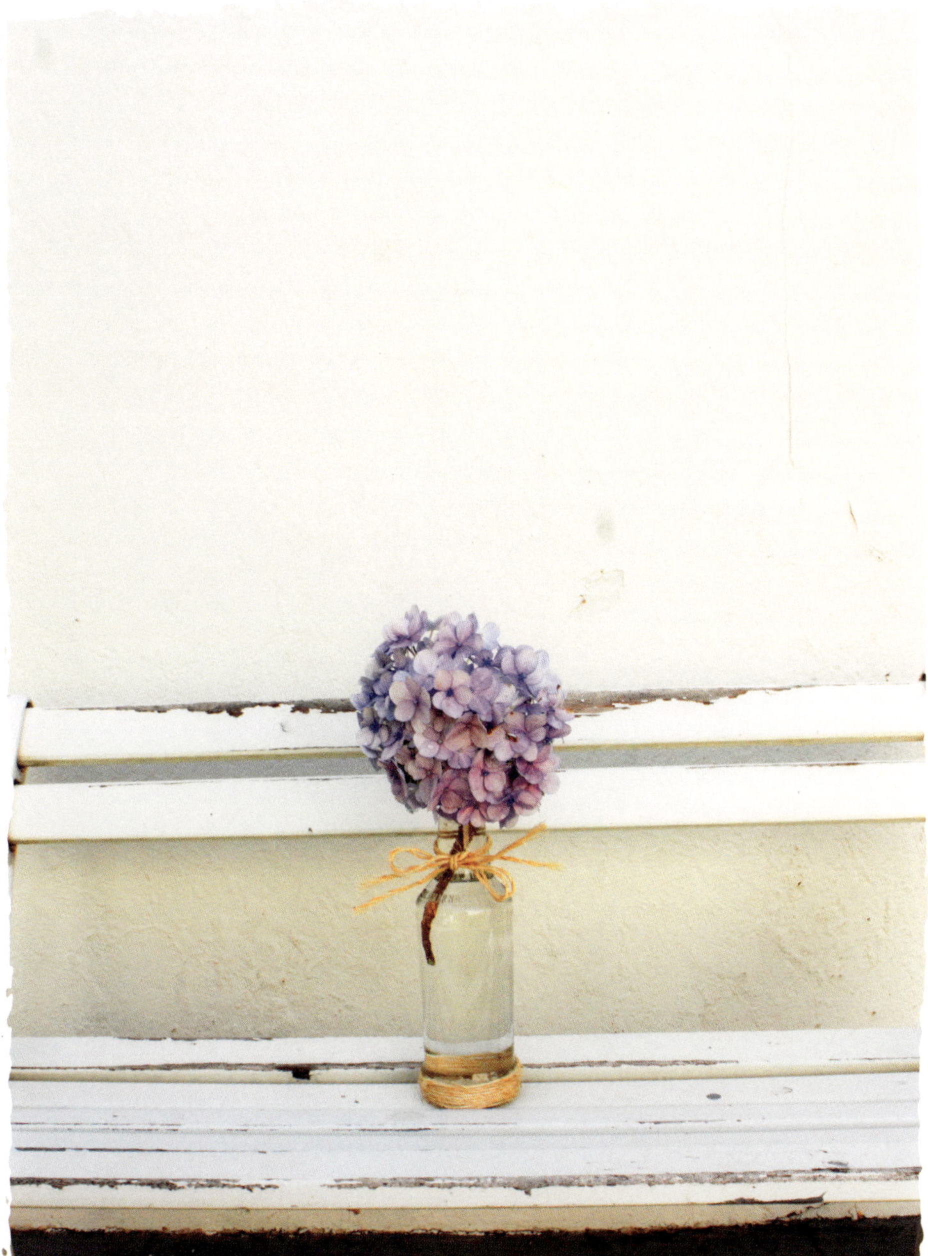

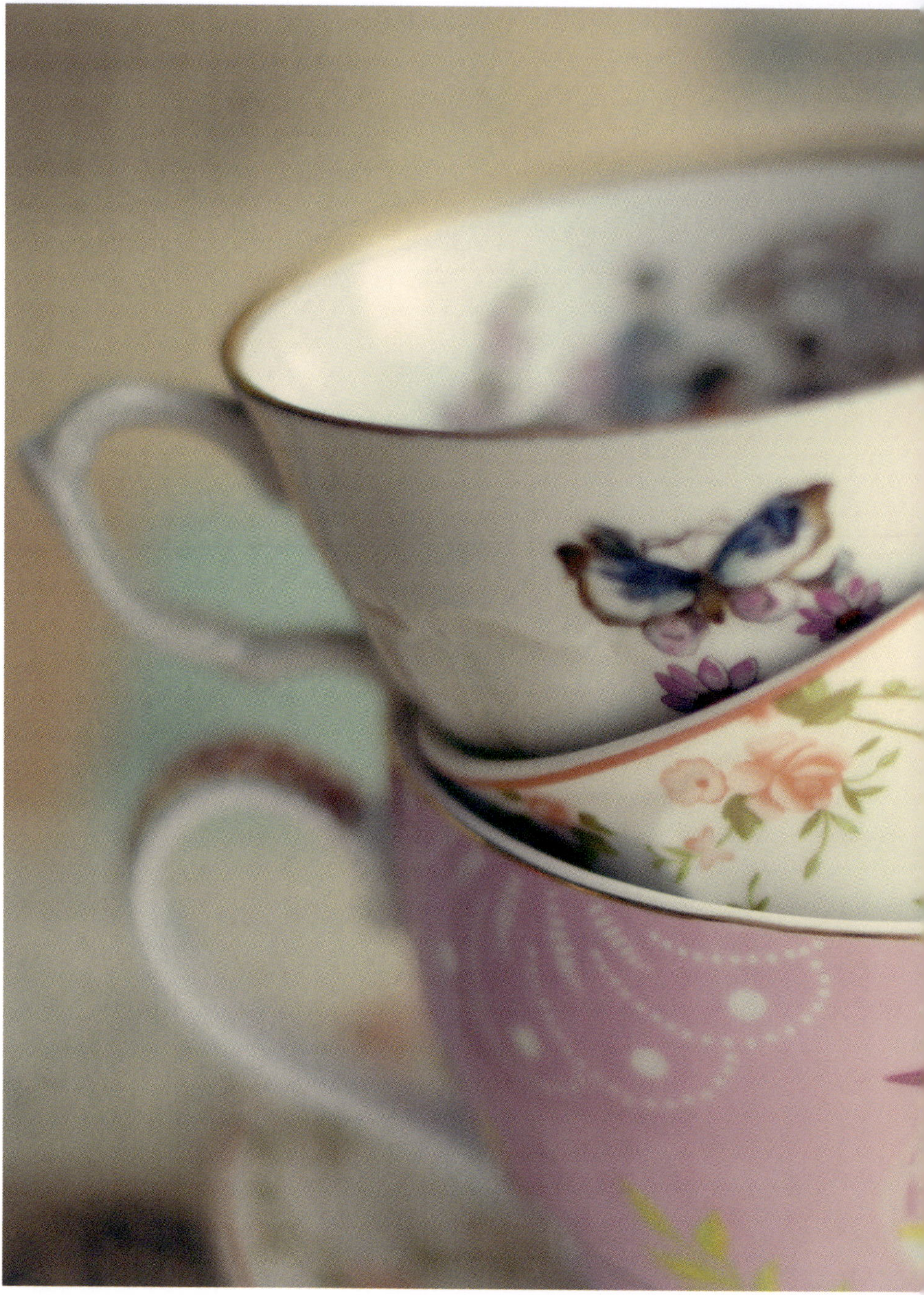

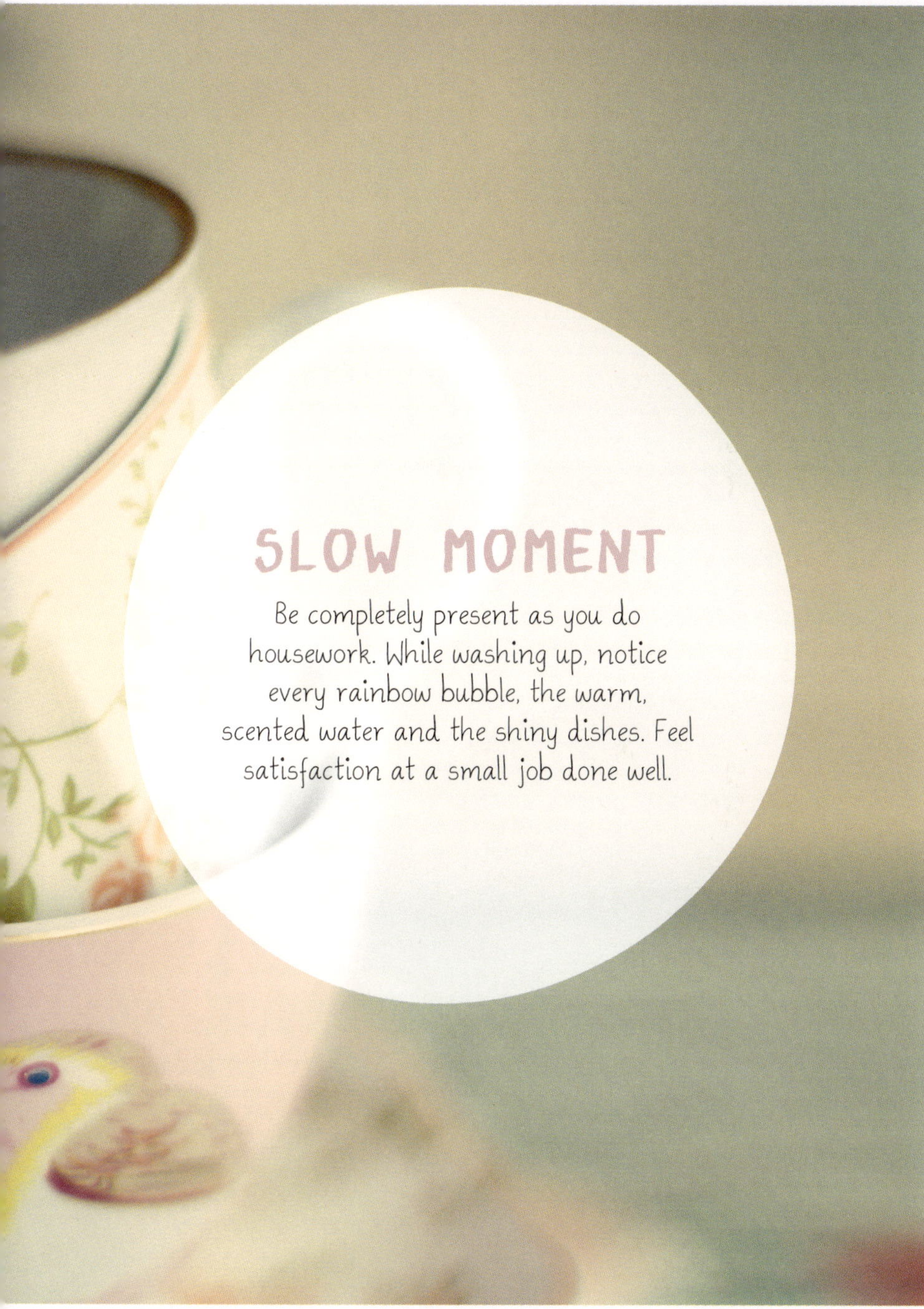

SLOW MOMENT

Be completely present as you do housework. While washing up, notice every rainbow bubble, the warm, scented water and the shiny dishes. Feel satisfaction at a small job done well.

THE JOY OF LIVING WITH LESS

Where does all this stuff come from? It can be very stressful when you look around your home and see stuff everywhere. Where on earth do you start? One way to make decluttering more enticing is to treat it like a game that everyone can get involved in. Get yourself a sack, laundry bin or a large, empty bag. Then choose a place to start – not a whole room, but just an area with clutter, such as shelves, a desk or worktop. Now count to 60 out loud and as you are doing so place the items in the bag that don't belong on the shelf or worktop. If you have finished one area before reaching 60, then move on to another. When the time's up, sort through the items in the bag and make one pile of keepers, one pile of rubbish and one pile for items that you can't accommodate. Then, return the keepers to their places, assigning a home to each one.

SUSTAINABLE LIVING

One of the key points of slow living is striving to live more sustainably and reduce our own carbon footprints, limiting conspicuous consumption and being more mindful of what we are buying. From the fabrics used to make our clothes to the methods used to grow our food, slow living asks us to make choices that will not only help us feel healthy, but will minimize our use of resources. As a consumer, you can do more by only purchasing products from ethical companies and ones that have sustainable production methods.

When you love what you have,
you have everything you need.

HOW TO RECONNECT AND STAY CONNECTED

SLOW RITUALS WITH FRIENDS AND FAMILY

Weekends and evenings can zip past in a blur of errands, appointments, homework and housework, and when you're on this survival-mode treadmill it can be difficult to find time for slow moments and the chance to reconnect with friends or family. One way to create this time is to form traditions and rituals – sacred slow moments and a chance to play – which are built into your calendar and are non-negotiable. Spending time together is comforting and creates bonds, and making it part of the weekly routine will benefit everyone, boosting self-esteem, resilience and a sense of belonging and security. Above all it's great fun and creates memories that last forever. Personalize your rituals to make them special to you.

When practising your new rituals, bear in mind the principles of slow:

- Let each person set their own pace – don't get impatient or hurry anyone along. Each person's needs are of equal importance.
- Be present and take notice of your friends and family members, connect and be fully in the moment – if you usually twitch at the sight of mess or a pile of washing up, try to block it out and keep the family ritual the priority.
- Just listen – often when we are listening to others speaking, we aren't really focusing on what they're saying because we're too busy thinking about what we're going to say next. Listen to the conversation and allow for a moment of silence before you speak.

Warning: these ideas do not include sitting together and zoning out on your phones and tablets. Switch them off and place them in a shoebox or somewhere out of sight to avoid temptation!

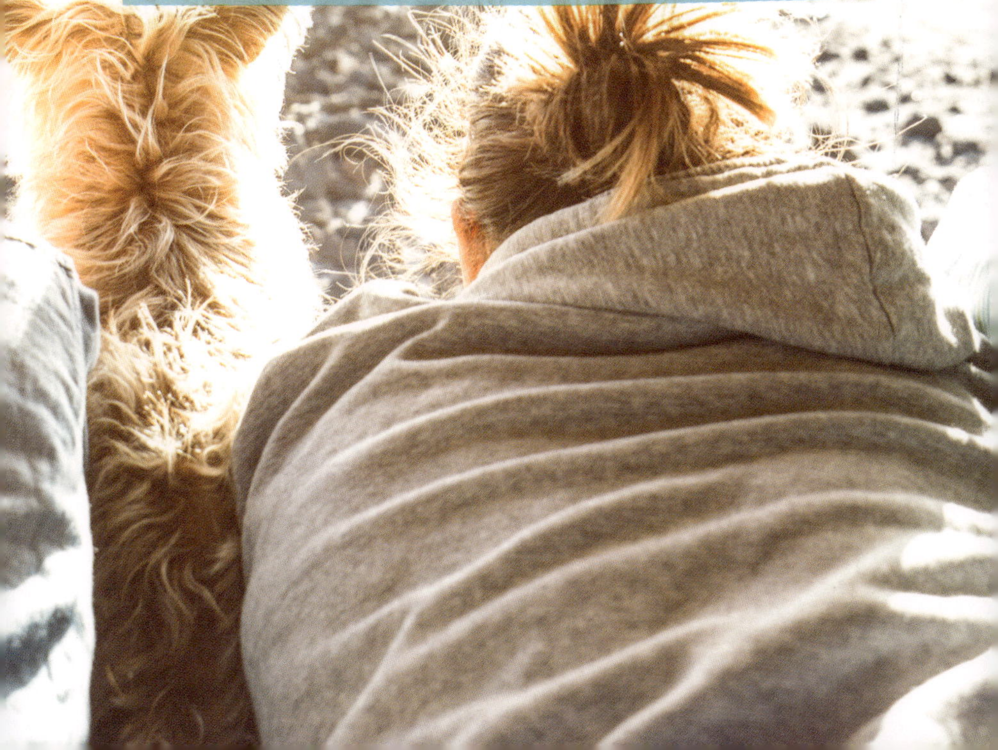

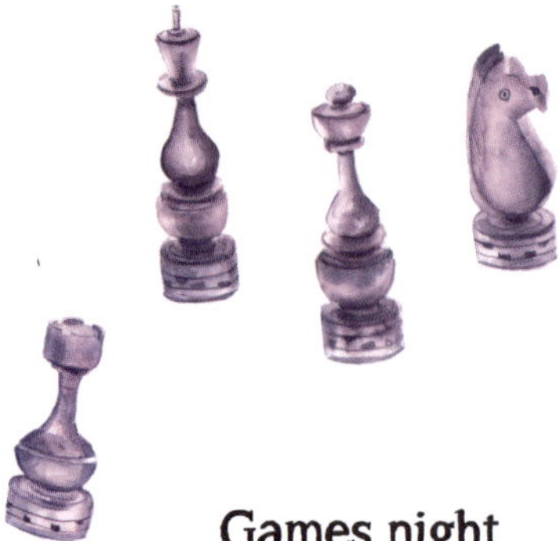

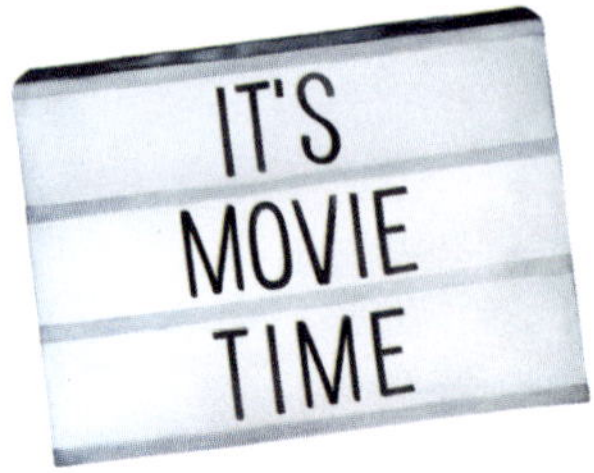

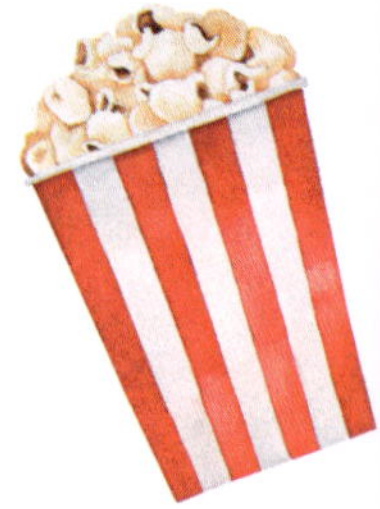

Games night

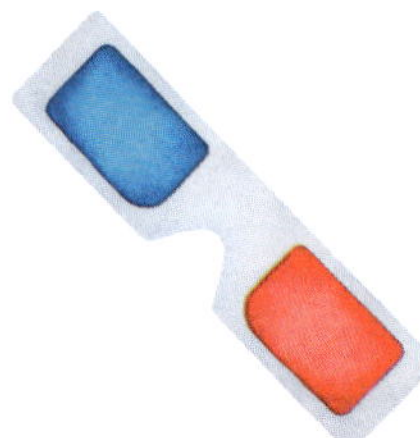

Pick a weeknight and get your brain working on problem-solving and strategy with a board or card game. Personalize the evening with some fun props – perhaps paint the nails of the winner, play hide-and-seek between games (just as fun for adults!), allow texting language in a game of Scrabble or set off party poppers when someone is released from jail in Monopoly.

Film night

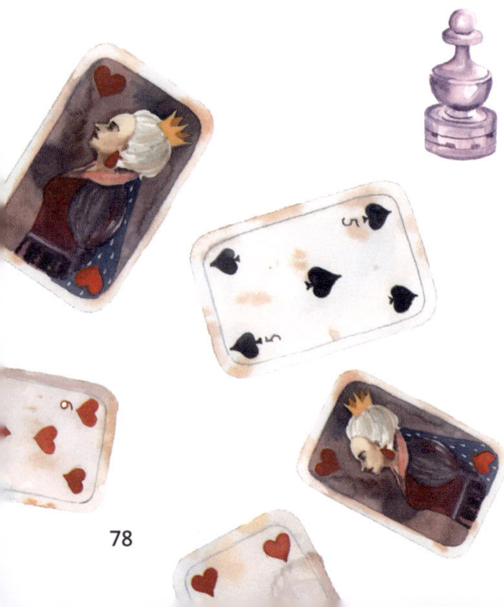

Pick a family-friendly film, light the fire and snuggle together on the sofa with a bowl of homemade popcorn. Make the evening more special by dressing up like the characters in the film, making a den out of furniture, cushions and blankets, turning out the lights and using candles instead, speaking in accents from characters in the film or making food that matches what you're watching – fondue or hotpot for a film set in snow, or mocktails for a film set on a desert island, for example.

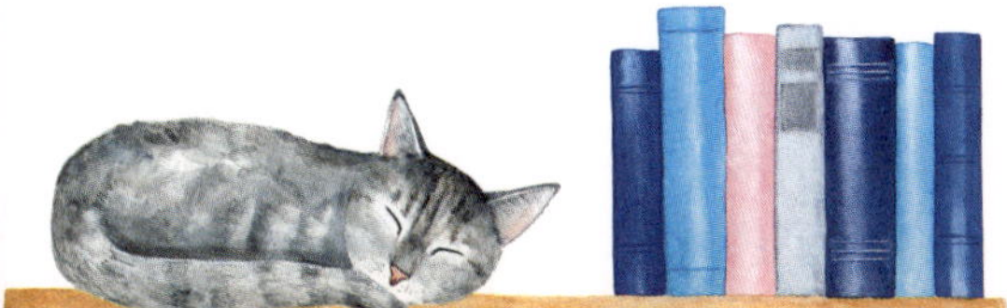

Book club

Not everyone likes to read, but reading aloud can make for a special ritual. This is something that people enjoy at any age – it promotes discussion and imaginative thinking as you discover a story and follow it together. The best stories challenge your perceptions, shape you and become part of you. Begin with the classics and make them age-appropriate, like *Little Women*, *Harry Potter and the Philosopher's Stone* or *A Wrinkle in Time* for younger ones or try some modern-day classics for adults, such as *The Book of Dust*, *The Power* or *When Breath Becomes Air*.

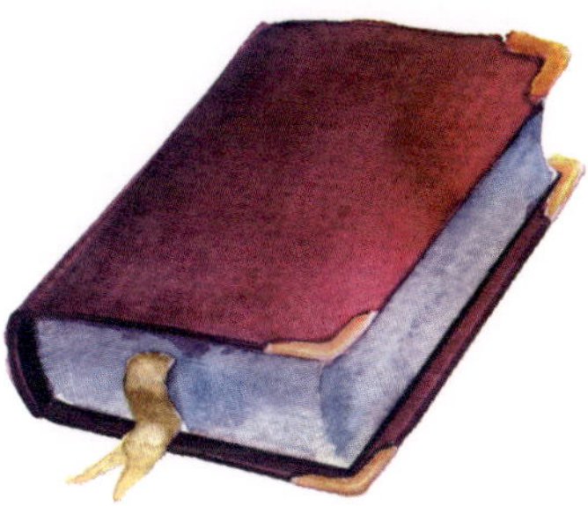

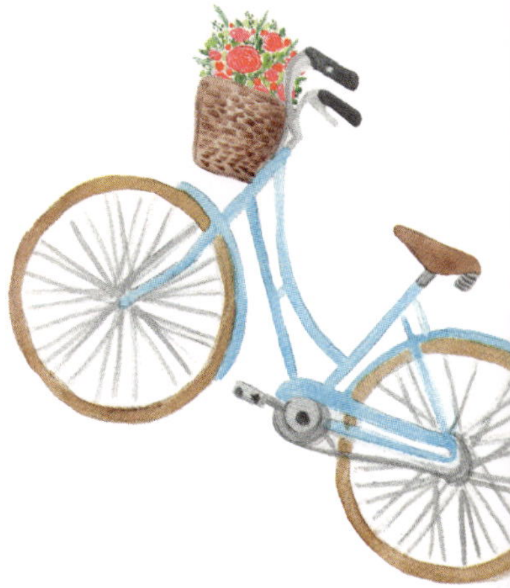

Green exercise

"Green exercise" is any physical activity you take part in outside, in natural surroundings. Take a leaf out of the Slow Bicycle Movement's remit and take to two wheels, sitting upright as you pootle through the countryside at a sedate 6 miles per hour. Just cruising allows you to see the world at a gentler pace and chat as you enjoy the ride. However, any form of exercise, be it a walk, a run or swim, for example, will provide a mood boost with the release of "happy" hormones, endorphins and dopamine.

Outdoor play

Take in a sunset on the beach, then enjoy an evening stargazing – wrap up warm, put blankets out, take a nighttime picnic and look up at the sky. If you have children, let them set the pace when you're in the great outdoors – if they're small, make mud pies, thread daisy chains, go bug hunting, climb trees, identify birds or simply kick a ball around. Encourage them to learn about plants by allocating a patch of ground in your garden to them – let them pick seeds to sow and help them to nurture their plants.

Children rule (just for an hour or two!)

Let your children spark their imagination – studies show that little ones with active imaginations are happier and more resilient when dealing with life's ups and downs. And besides, they spend nearly every day following rules and timetables, so it's a great way to teach them to be responsible for their own decision-making. Encourage them to think beyond expensive excursions by providing a small budget to allow for going swimming or buying ingredients to make a cake.

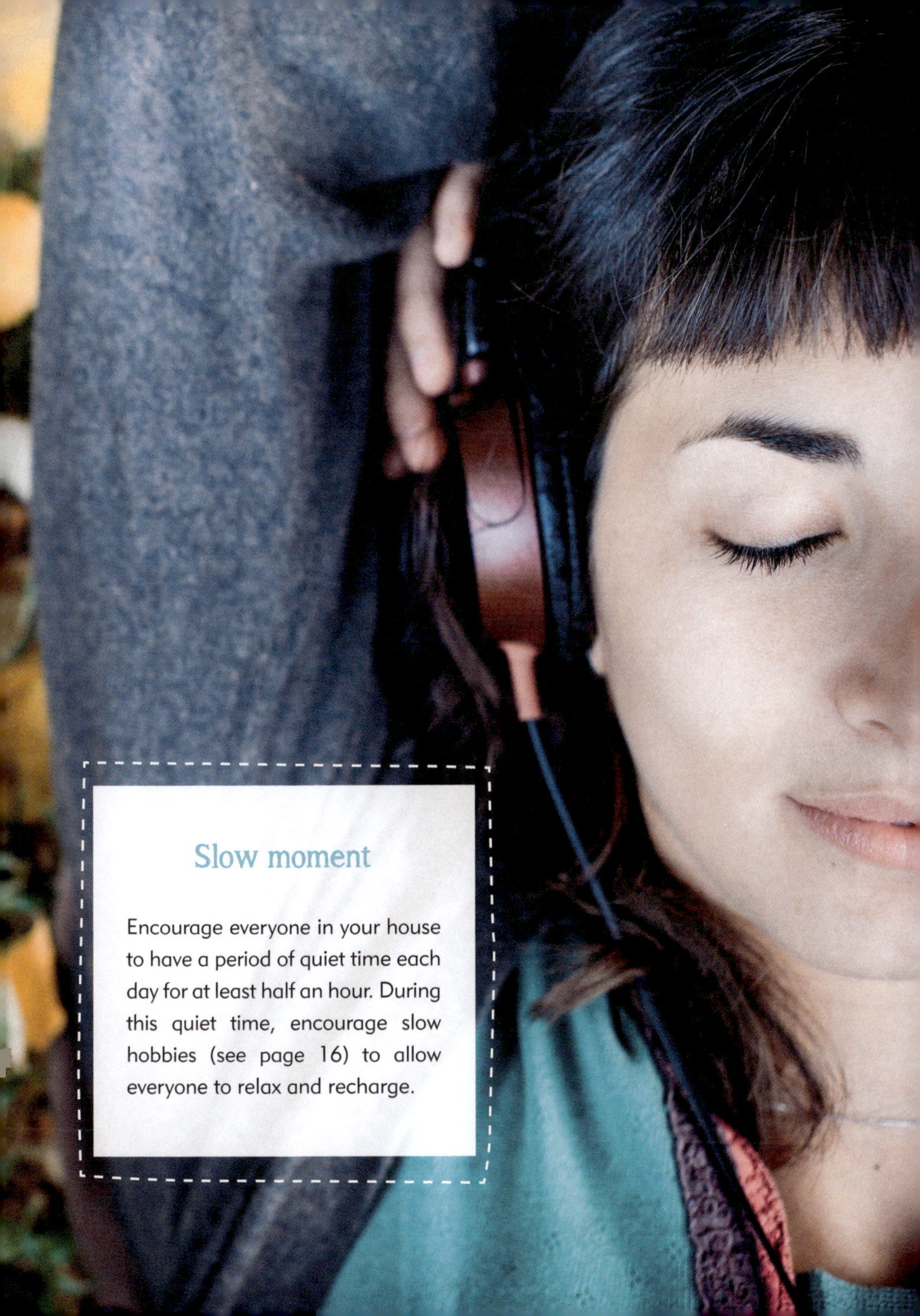

Slow moment

Encourage everyone in your house to have a period of quiet time each day for at least half an hour. During this quiet time, encourage slow hobbies (see page 16) to allow everyone to relax and recharge.

LITTLE DAILY SLOW RITUALS

Get up half an hour early, make a hot drink and take it back to bed

Give your loved ones a kiss before you head out of the house in the morning

Cloud-watch

Watch the shadows on the ground

Open the windows and listen to the birds

Stroke your pet

Ask your loved ones about their day

Spend half an hour sketching, doodling or colouring in

Have a cuddle

Dance to your favourite song

Lie on the floor and stretch out

Write a postcard to a friend or family member

Light a candle at dinner time

Walk round your neighbourhood

Make a cup of tea and watch the world go by

Admire flowers

Tuck your children into bed

Walk round the garden and notice what's growing

Meditate

Read a chapter of a book before bed

RECIPE FOR A SLOW WEEKEND (OR WELL-EARNED DAYS OFF)

Welcome the morning into your home

Open your curtains or shutters, fold back your sheets and open a window in your bedroom to let in the fresh morning air – but not for too long if it's chilly!

Take a trip

Leave your camera at home, place your phone in your bag or pocket and only take it out when you absolutely need to. Get the most out of the experience by bringing your presence and full attention to all that you experience. Savour the sights, sounds and smells of your new location.

Travel to a local market or shop

Pick up eggs and oranges for breakfast. Squeeze the oranges and add ice cubes to create your own juice. Or if it's winter...

... make a batch of porridge

Hot and nourishing, porridge is a wholesome and delicious start to the day. Decorate your bowl with your favourite seasonal toppings, such as apples or blackberries.

Bake bread for lunch

A simple round of white bread takes no longer than 1 hour and 20 minutes to prepare and prove and just 30 minutes baking time in a normal oven. The smell of it baking can lift your heart as you…

… act like a cat

Cats are true artists of slow living and they know well the power of curling up in a patch of sunlight. Find your own sunlight and settle into it. You don't have to do anything other than mindfully enjoy yourself; note the warmth of the sun on your skin and the texture of the rug or blanket against your bare feet.

Make a pilgrimage

Go to your nearest spot of nature, whether it is the coast or a little wooded copse. If you live in a city, head to the park or a nearby beach or lake.

Make yourself lunch

Cut thick slices of the bread you baked to dip into soup made with seasonal vegetables, or pile it with cold salted butter and crumbly cheese.

Start a small crafting project

Maybe you've been inspired by your morning walk. What colours, shapes or textures did you find in nature that might inspire you to create?

Create your own flavoured cooking oils

Simmer olive oil with a quantity of flavouring and bottle in a sterile jar.

Prepare dinner

Play a board game

Enlist your friends and family to join in. It will gently stretch your mind and give you something to talk and laugh over.

Light candles

As evening falls, light candles to fill your home with gentle light.

SIMPLIFY YOUR CALENDAR

JOMO

the joy of missing out

Slow living is living purposefully, mindfully and happily. Sometimes this comes from saying "yes" to the things we love and spending the extra time to really relish an activity or time with someone special. However, time and "yes" are not infinite resources. Sometimes we must choose to miss out on an activity that we do not have time for and this decision is often accompanied by a feeling of guilt. You may even assume that a more accomplished person would find a way to juggle everything. Release yourself from that guilt and embrace JOMO, the joy of missing out. Learn to trust your decisions; time is your most precious resource and you are right to not spend it on activities you don't want to do or are unable to dedicate your full attention to. Instead of feeling guilty about spending an evening replenishing your energy, try to experience joy in making the right decision for you, your body and your health.

JONO

the joy of no

You can't experience all the benefits of JOMO without first engaging with JONO, or the joy of no. Move past thinking of "no" as a negative or limiting word. Think of it instead as your key to freedom. Replenishing your energy through relaxation or single-tasking an activity that is important to you is a worthy and necessary action. Try to keep this in your mind as you say "no" to a potential engagement and speak with confidence. It's only human to feel regret at missing out on an activity you had wanted to take part in, and do express your regrets where necessary, but let go of your guilt.

less is more

DOWNSIZE YOUR CALENDAR

You may have trouble embracing JOMO if you feel as though you are exchanging doing something for doing nothing. Allocate time to yourself on a regular basis and block out time on your calendar as "me time" – to just do the things that you enjoy or to sit and think or meditate and appreciate your own company. Then you have a "me" plan to fall back on when saying "no" to an activity.

QUALITY NOT QUANTITY

Try doing less in terms of how much you commit to, such as clubs and engagements, and even subscriptions to magazines and blogs. Restrict to a handful of the ones that enrich your life rather than ones that you feel burdened by. This will not only reduce your stress levels but ultimately make your experiences more satisfying.

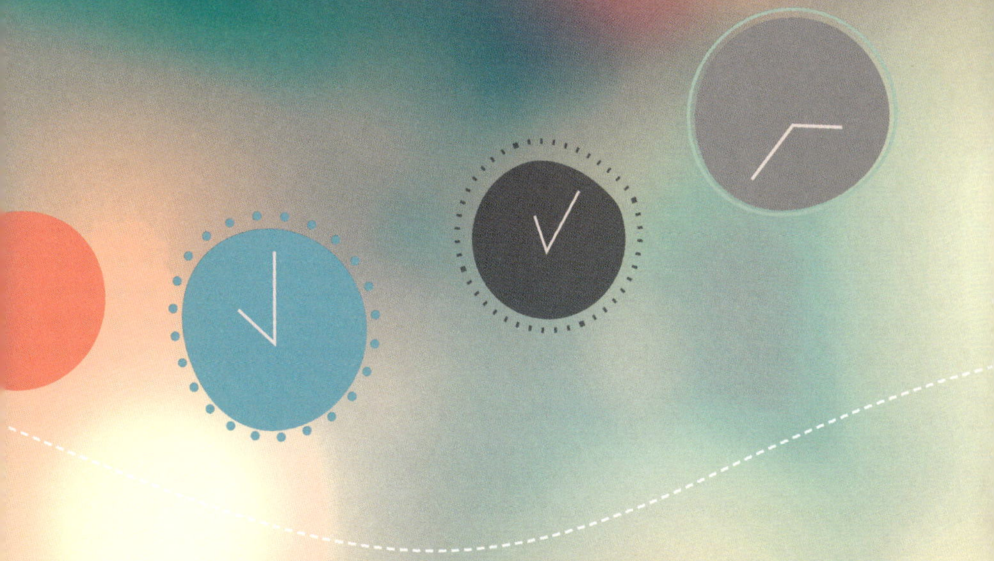

Schedule more in-between time

Life can feel like an endless list of appointments and responsibilities as you go seamlessly from one to the next. Slow this right down by scheduling in more wiggle room between activities, so if you normally allow 10 minutes to go from one engagement to the next, schedule in 20 minutes instead.

SLOW FOOD

WHAT IS SLOW FOOD?

The concept of slow living was first coined at the formation of the Slow Food movement. Their values are about maintaining ethical, healthy and sustainable practices in food production and defending gastronomic traditions on a global scale. Following this movement as an individual extends to buying seasonal and local produce and cooking food from scratch rather than eating ready meals, which contain preservatives and where some of the content may be of questionable origin. Preparing fresh, homemade meals also offers the opportunity to really savour the cooking process – first finding a recipe or picking a few simple, healthy ingredients and allowing your culinary skills to guide you. Cooking can be very companionable, and it is a pleasant way to spend time with friends or family.

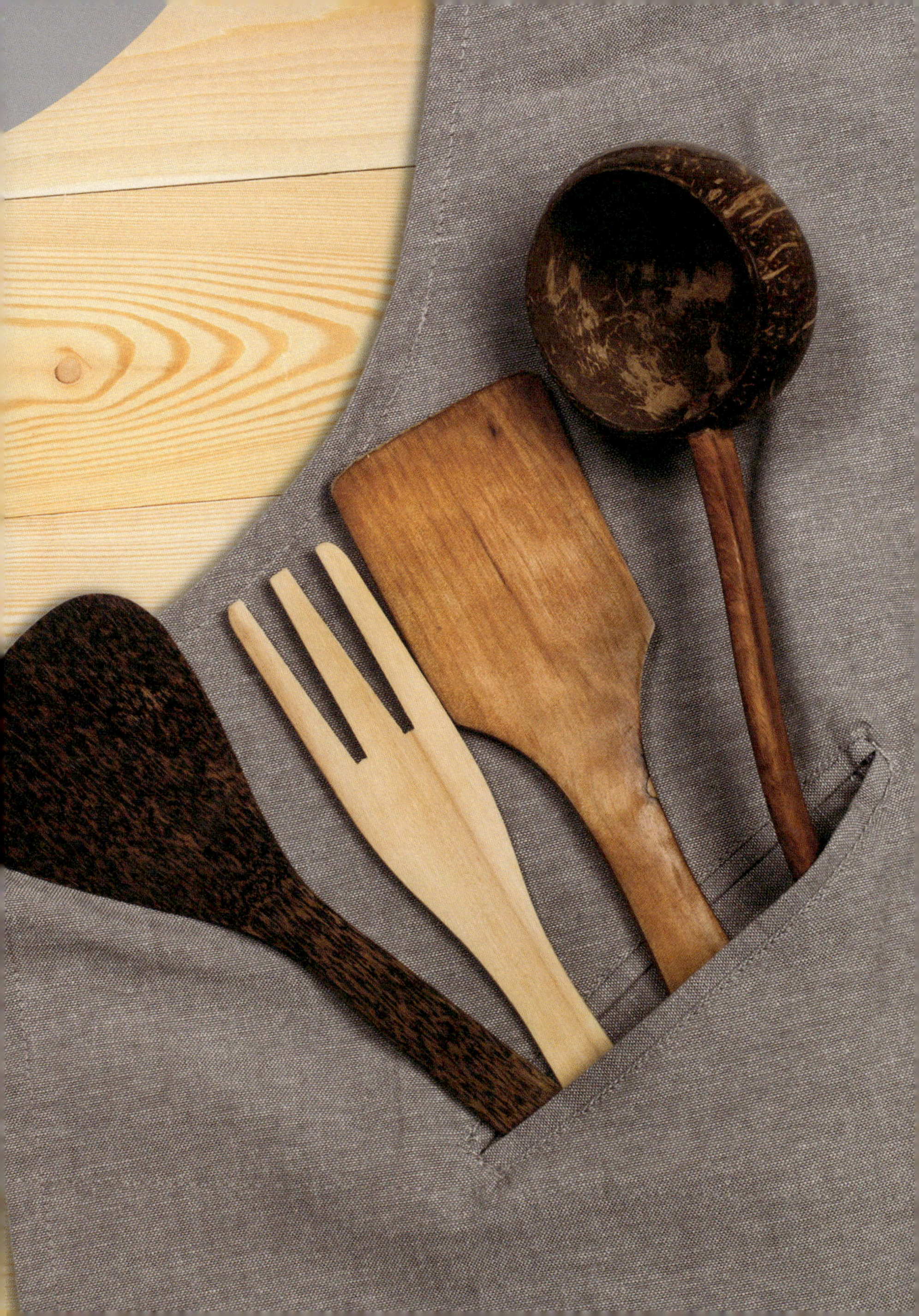

EAT MORE SLOWLY

It sounds like the sort of thing your mum used to say when you were small and wolfing down your food so you could carry on playing, but there are some major health benefits to taking your time to chew your food.

Eating slowly has enormous benefits to health and, conversely, according to research in Japan, gobbling down your food leads to an increased risk of heart attack, stroke and diabetes. It only takes a few minutes longer to chew your food properly, and it reduces stress on the body and you enjoy your food more. The other main benefits include:

Weight loss (and keeping weight off)

A growing number of studies confirm that just by eating more slowly, you will consume fewer calories. The reason for this is that it takes approximately 20 minutes for our brains to become aware that we are full. Eating quickly results in eating beyond the point when we are full. Obviously it also depends on what you are eating as to whether you maintain a healthy weight.

Eating becomes a pleasure

It's difficult to enjoy your food if you're eating it quickly. Savour each mouthful and don't treat eating as another stressful task to be rushed and shoehorned between other stressful tasks.

Most of us enjoy eating foods that are deemed bad for us, so next time you want a sugar fix, eat just a small amount. A single square of good quality dark chocolate eaten slowly so that it melts in the mouth can be a superb treat, with the added benefit of offering a vitamin C hit and an antioxidant cleanse.

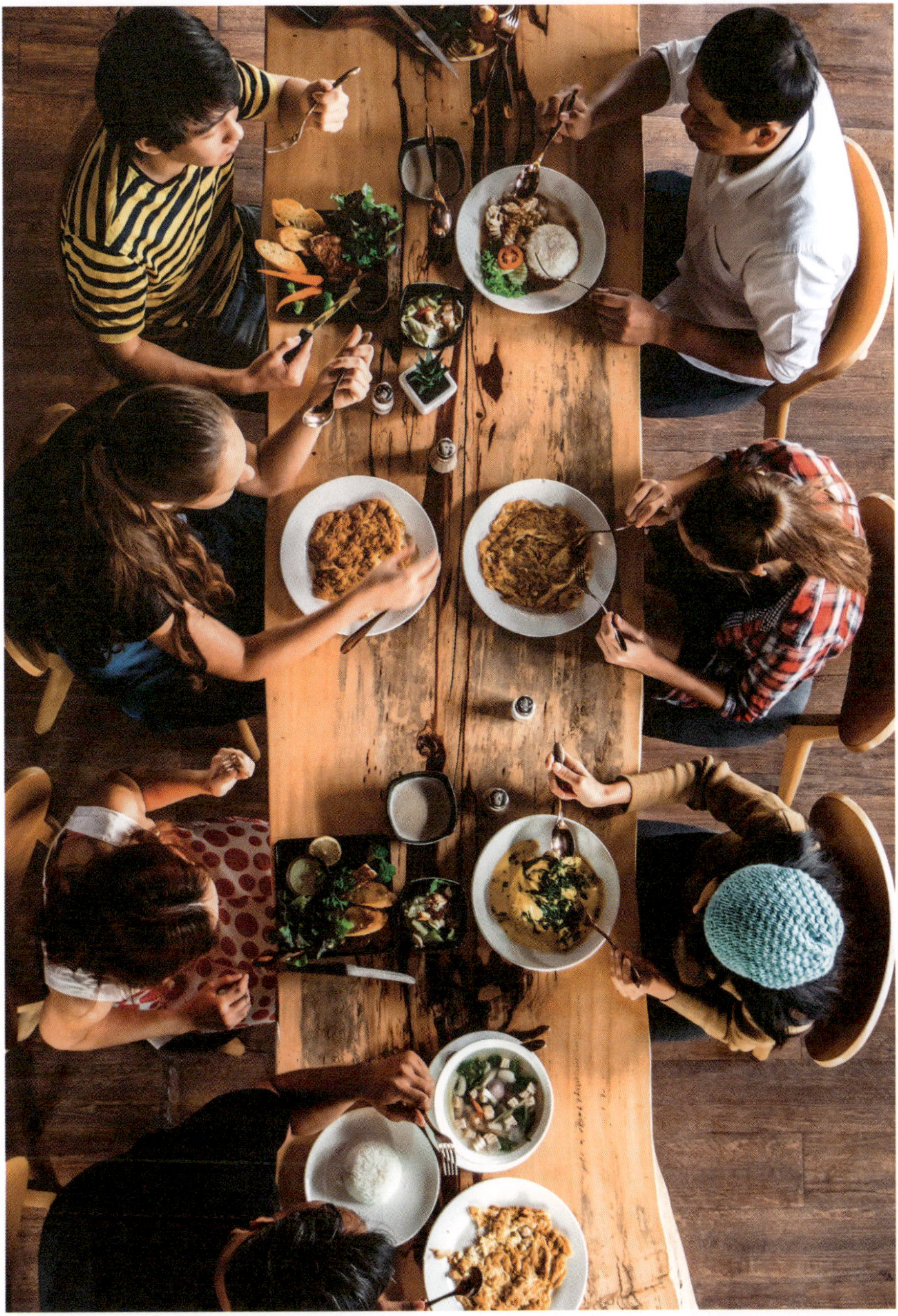

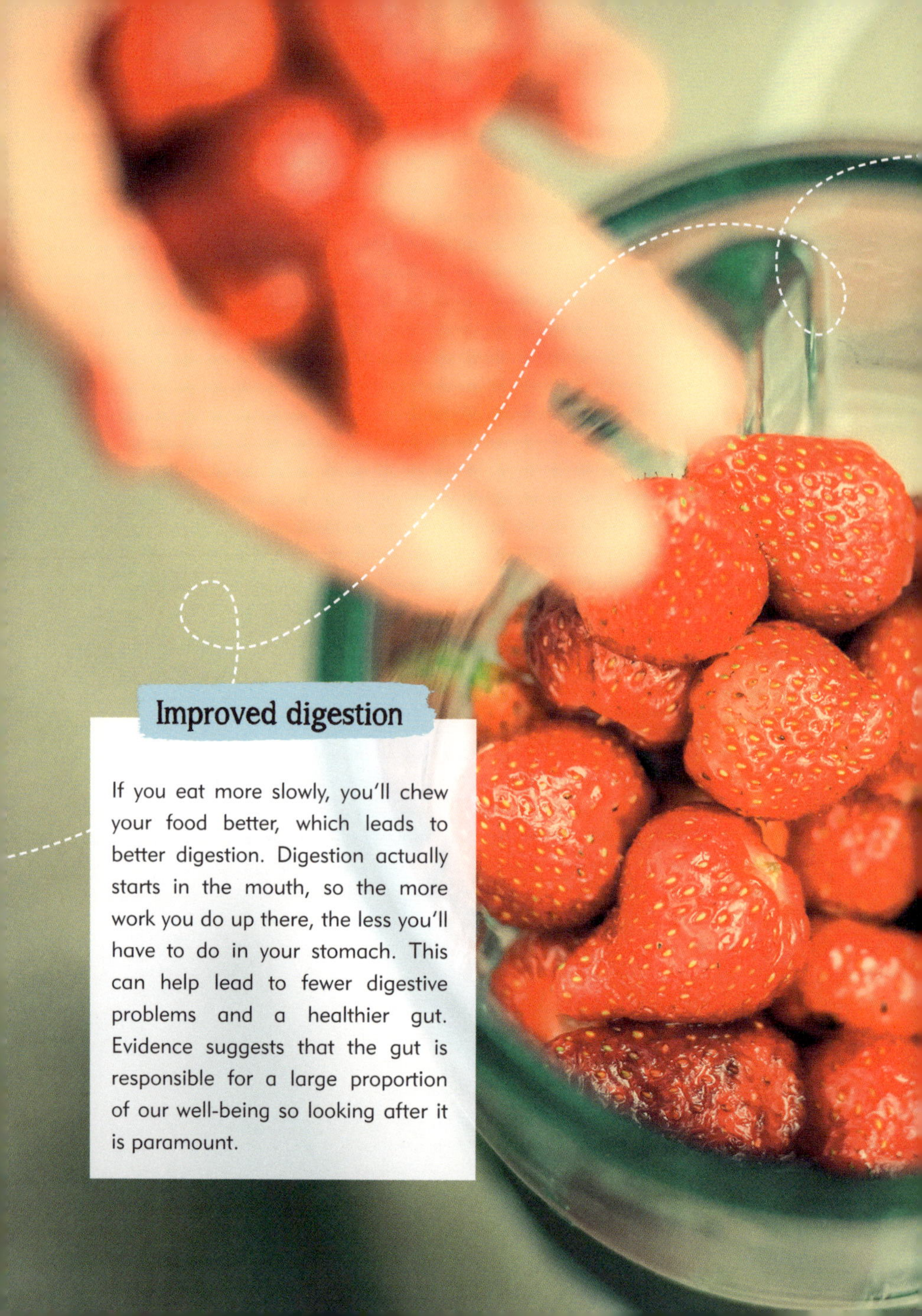

Improved digestion

If you eat more slowly, you'll chew your food better, which leads to better digestion. Digestion actually starts in the mouth, so the more work you do up there, the less you'll have to do in your stomach. This can help lead to fewer digestive problems and a healthier gut. Evidence suggests that the gut is responsible for a large proportion of our well-being so looking after it is paramount.

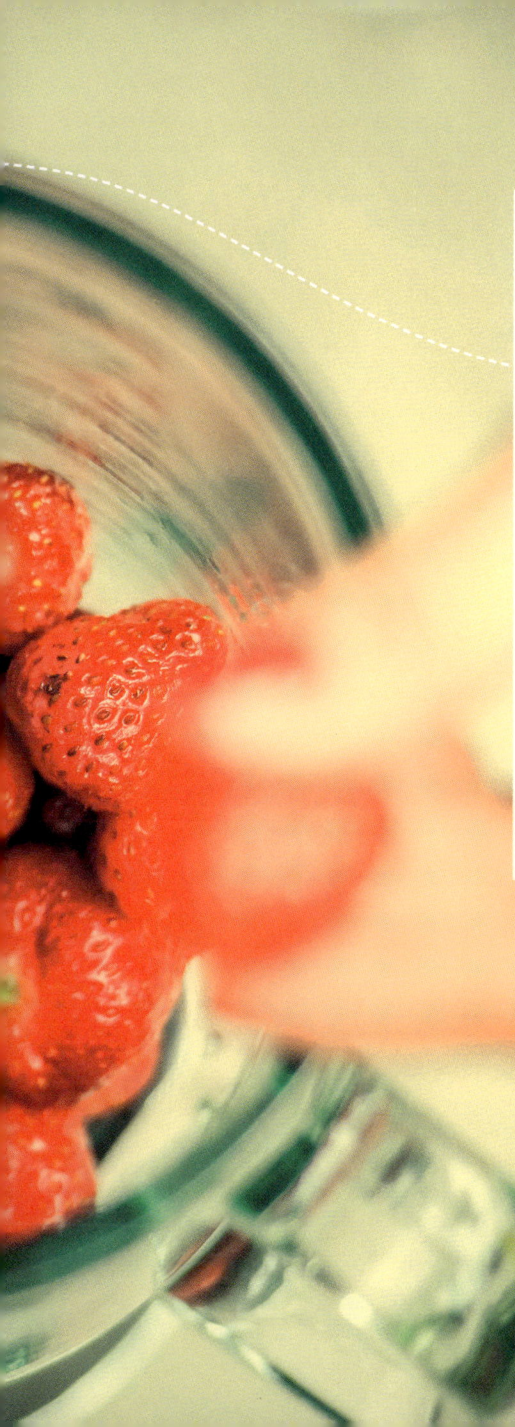

Lowered stress levels

Eating slowly, and paying attention to our eating, can be treated like a mindfulness exercise. As you eat your meal, focus all your attention on the tastes, sounds, smells and sensations you are experiencing, rather than anything else going on around you. See if turning the TV or radio off and eating in silence makes you appreciate the food and the feeling of being full more than usual. Try placing your fork down in-between mouthfuls and chewing each mouthful slowly in order to relish every taste sensation. Learn to view eating as a calming experience.

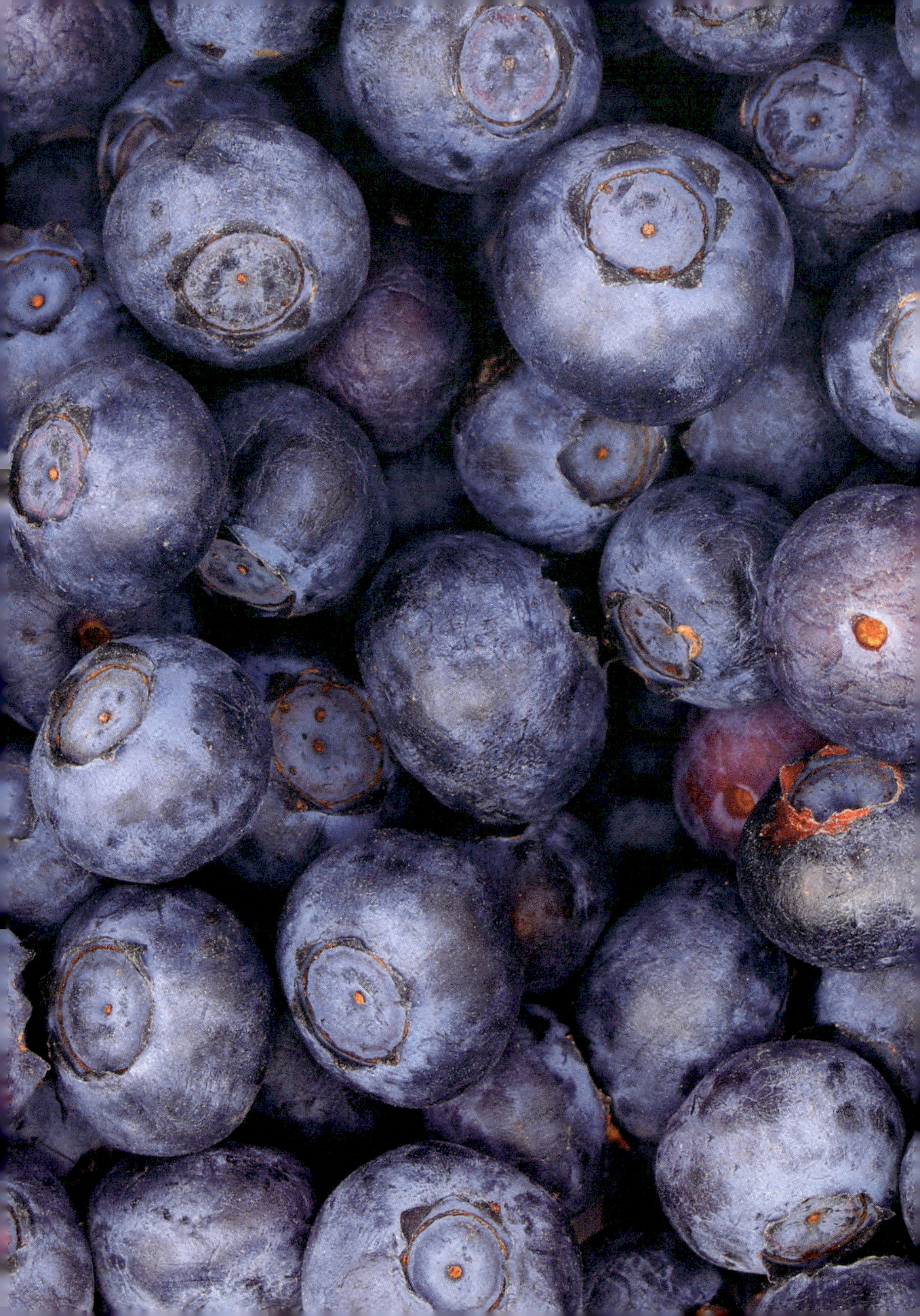

EAT FOODS THAT ENERGIZE YOU

Slow living often inspires a move towards healthier eating habits. Purposefully slowing down allows us to make more considered choices about what we put in our bodies in order to be healthier.

On the following pages are some simple meals that are fun to make and energizing to eat.

OVERNIGHT OATS

SERVES ONE

Spare jam jars really come into their own with this delicious breakfast. It's super-simple to make and keeps for up to four days, so you can make a small batch each time.

PREPARATION TIME:

5 minutes

COOKING TIME:

None, but must be left overnight in the fridge

INGREDIENTS:

100 ml (3½ fl oz) milk (dairy, soya or nut)
100 g (3½ oz) porridge oats
100 ml (3½ fl oz) natural yoghurt
1 tsp chia seeds
Optional extras:
Pumpkin seeds, sunflower seeds, a spoonful of nut butter, flaked nuts, granola, honey
Topping suggestions:
Banana, berries, coconut flakes

METHOD

Add the ingredients to a clean jam jar (or other glass jar) and mix it together.

Close the lid and place in the fridge overnight. You'll find that the chia seeds have absorbed the liquid in the morning and they taste delicious!

Add some mashed-up banana, berries or other toppings before eating.

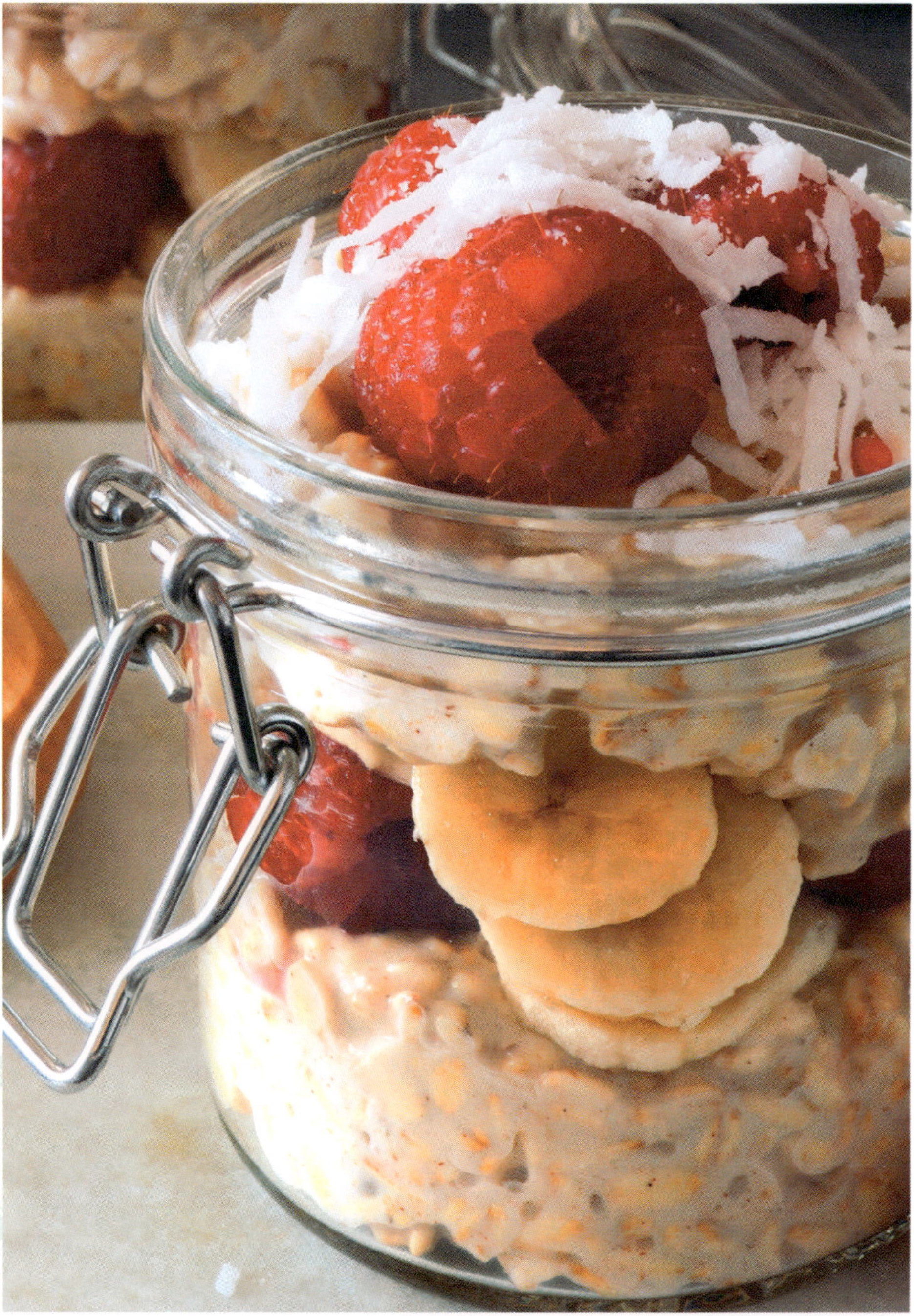

RAW ENERGY FUDGE

MAKES 16 SQUARES

This recipe makes around 16 squares, enough to provide you with snacks throughout the week. Eschew over-packaged and over-processed confectionery and enjoy these chocolatey fudge bites from your kitchen.

PREPARATION TIME:
15 minutes

COOKING TIME:
No cooking, but 3 hours chilling

INGREDIENTS:
150 g (5¼ oz) sesame seeds
4 tbsp coconut oil
60 g (2 oz) raw cacao powder
2 tbsp carob powder
100 ml (3½ fl oz) agave syrup

METHOD

Blend the sesame seeds on a high speed in a food processor until finely ground. Melt the oil and add, with the remaining ingredients, to the sesame seeds. Blend until fully combined.

Pour into a 30 x 23 cm (12 x 9 in.) baking tray lined with baking paper and press down.

Chill for 2–3 hours until firm.

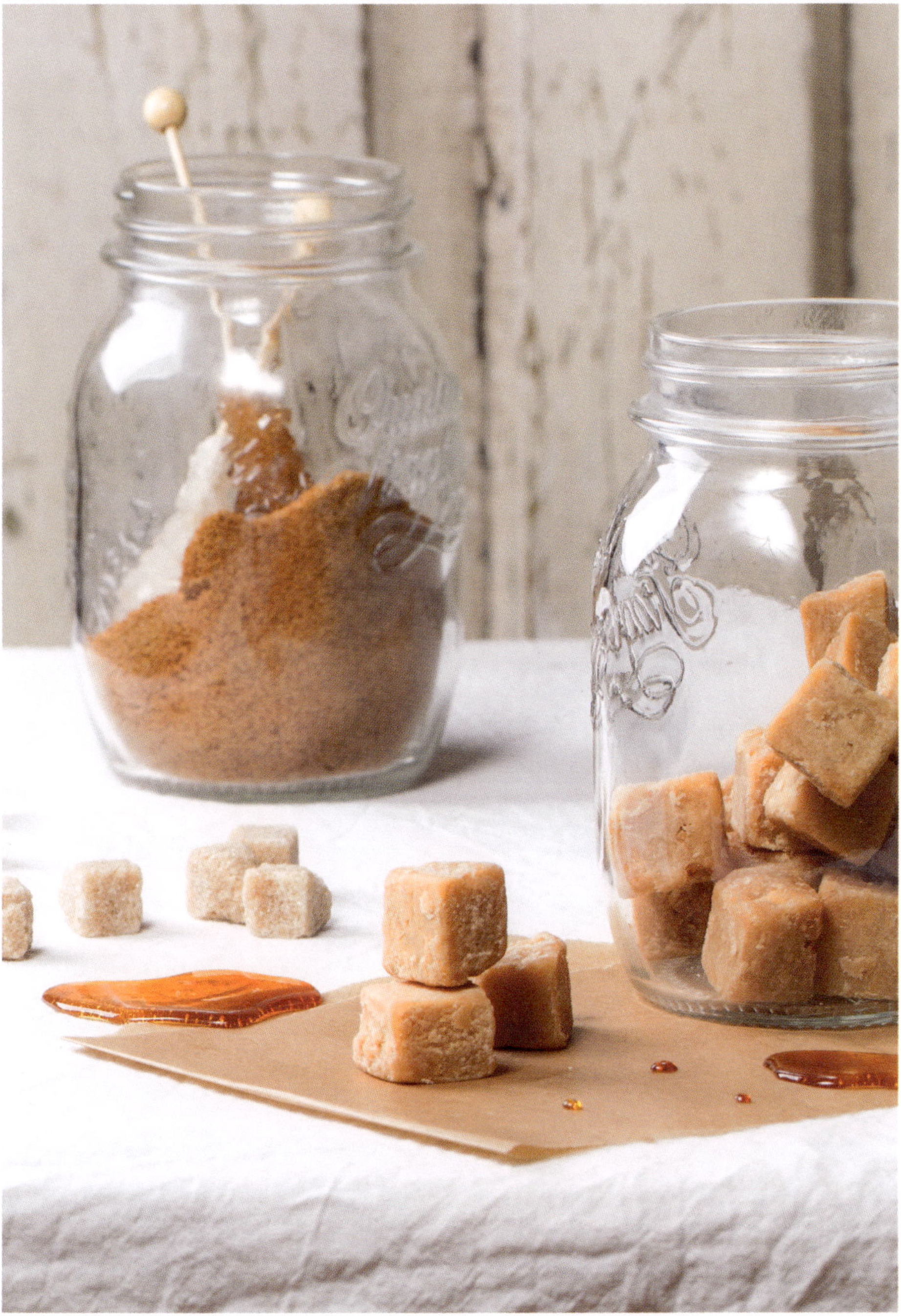

RAW ENERGY BALLS

MAKES 15 BALLS

You'll get around 15 small but mighty balls from this recipe. Full of natural sugars, protein and fibre, they'll boost you throughout your day.

PREPARATION TIME:

15 minutes

COOKING TIME:

No cooking, but 15 minutes chilling

INGREDIENTS:

220 g (7¾ oz) dates
3 tbsp peanut butter
55 g (2 oz) dark chocolate
1 tbsp ground flax seeds
160 g (5½ oz) rolled oats
40 g (1½ oz) almonds

METHOD

Grate the chocolate or break it into squares, depending on whether you'd prefer chocolate chips or an even chocolatey flavour.

Pulse together all of the ingredients in a blender until they make a thick paste.

Roll into spheres the size of ping-pong balls.

They are ready to eat straight away but 15 minutes in the fridge will help firm up the mixture. The perfect compromise is to snack on one while the rest cool in the fridge.

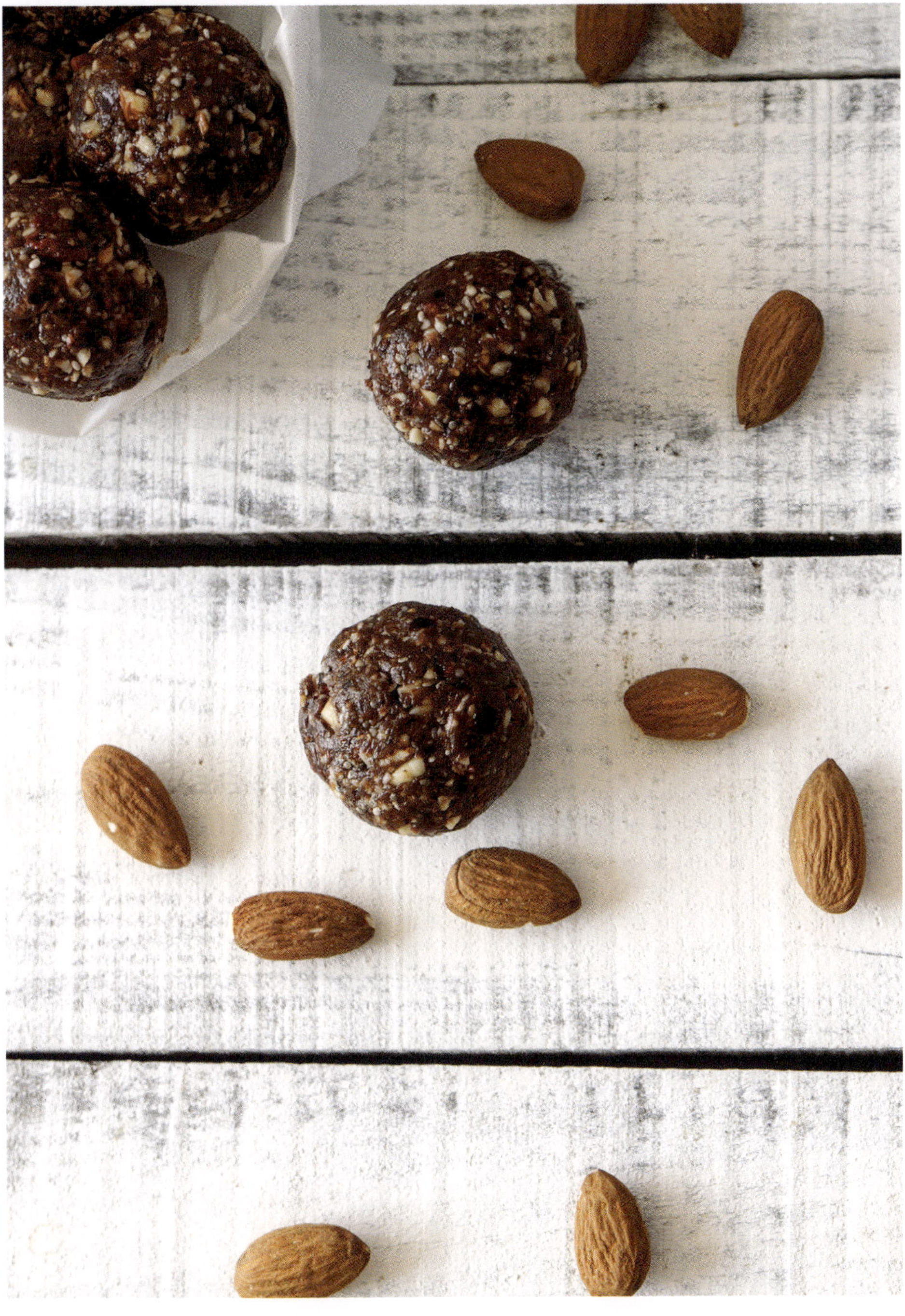

ELDERFLOWER FRITTERS

SERVES FIVE

This fragrant, summery treat makes a delicious dessert. Be sure to pluck the heads when the buds have just flowered for the best flavour.

PREPARATION TIME:
20 minutes

COOKING TIME:
2 minutes per head

INGREDIENTS:

15 elderflower heads
100 g (3½ oz) plain flour
2 tbsp oil, plus a pan of oil for frying
175 ml (6 fl oz) sparkling water
Cold plate of caster sugar
Honey or ice cream to serve

METHOD

Cut the elderflower heads so there is enough stem to hold them by. Shake off any little bugs and rinse them in cold water.

Sift the flour into a bowl and stir in the oil and water.

Heat the pan of oil until it sizzles when you flick a tiny drop of water into it.

Hold the elderflowers by their stems and dunk them into the batter mix, then push them headfirst into the oil.

Fry for 1–2 minutes until batter is golden and crisp, then hold them first on some kitchen roll to soak the excess oil and then on the plate of caster sugar.

Serve hot with ice cream or a drizzle of honey.

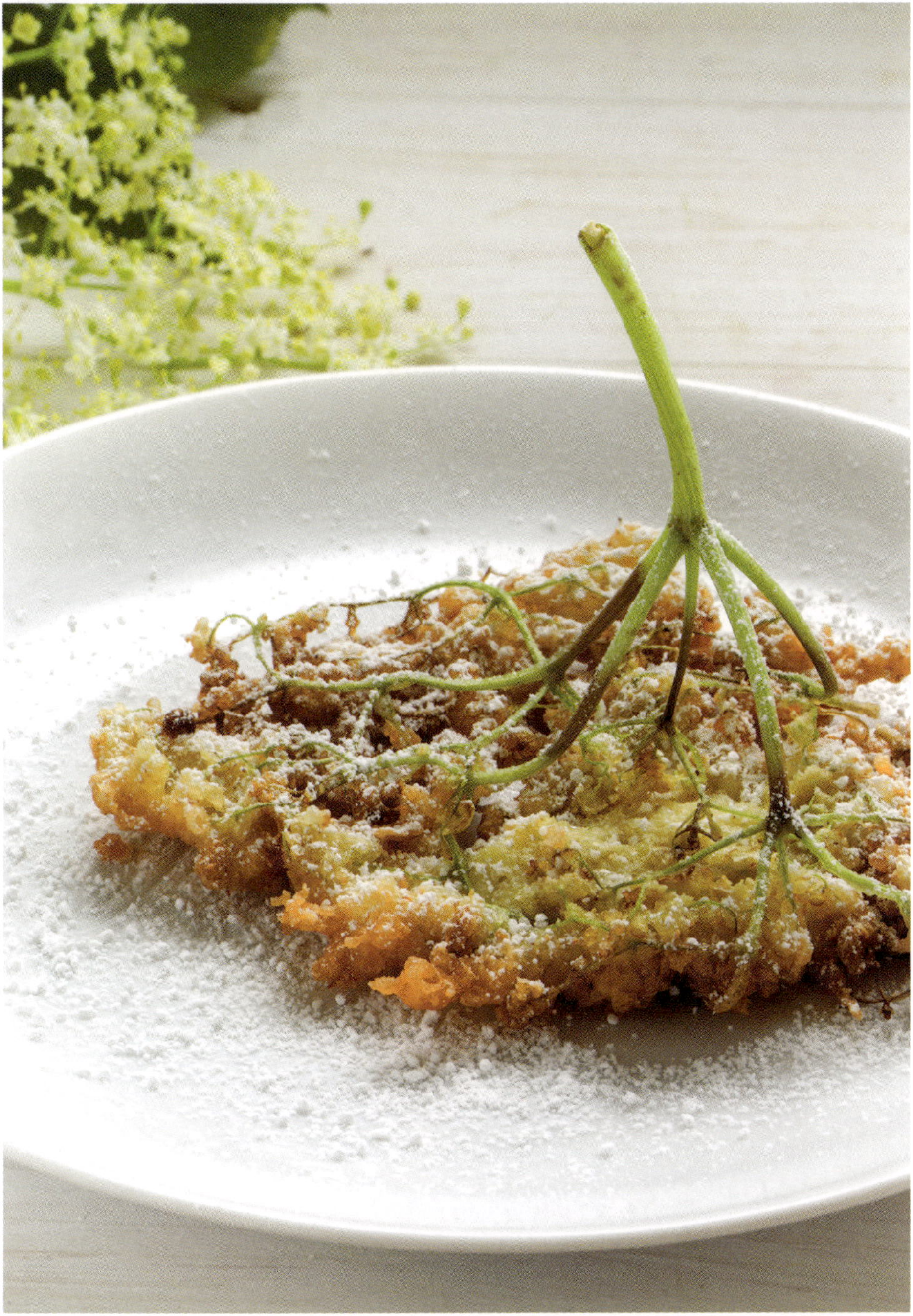

FORAGED WILD GARLIC PESTO

MAKES ONE JAR

The first crop of chives will be ready just as wild garlic is really coming into its own in spring. Combine the two for a fresh-tasting – and frankly quite powerful – homemade pesto. Thoroughly wash the wild garlic after you pick it and ensure it is dry before storing it in the fridge ahead of making this recipe.

PREPARATION TIME:
15 minutes

COOKING TIME:
None

INGREDIENTS:
1 large bunch wild garlic
150 g (5¼ oz) chives
50 g (1¾ oz) pine nuts
150 ml (5 fl oz) olive oil
60 g (2 oz) Parmesan
Salt and black pepper
1 tbsp lemon juice

METHOD

Blitz the garlic, chives, pine nuts and olive oil in a blender until well-combined but still a little rough. Add more oil if you'd like the consistency to be smoother.

Add the cheese, salt and pepper to taste. Stir in the lemon juice just before serving, or at the end if making to store.

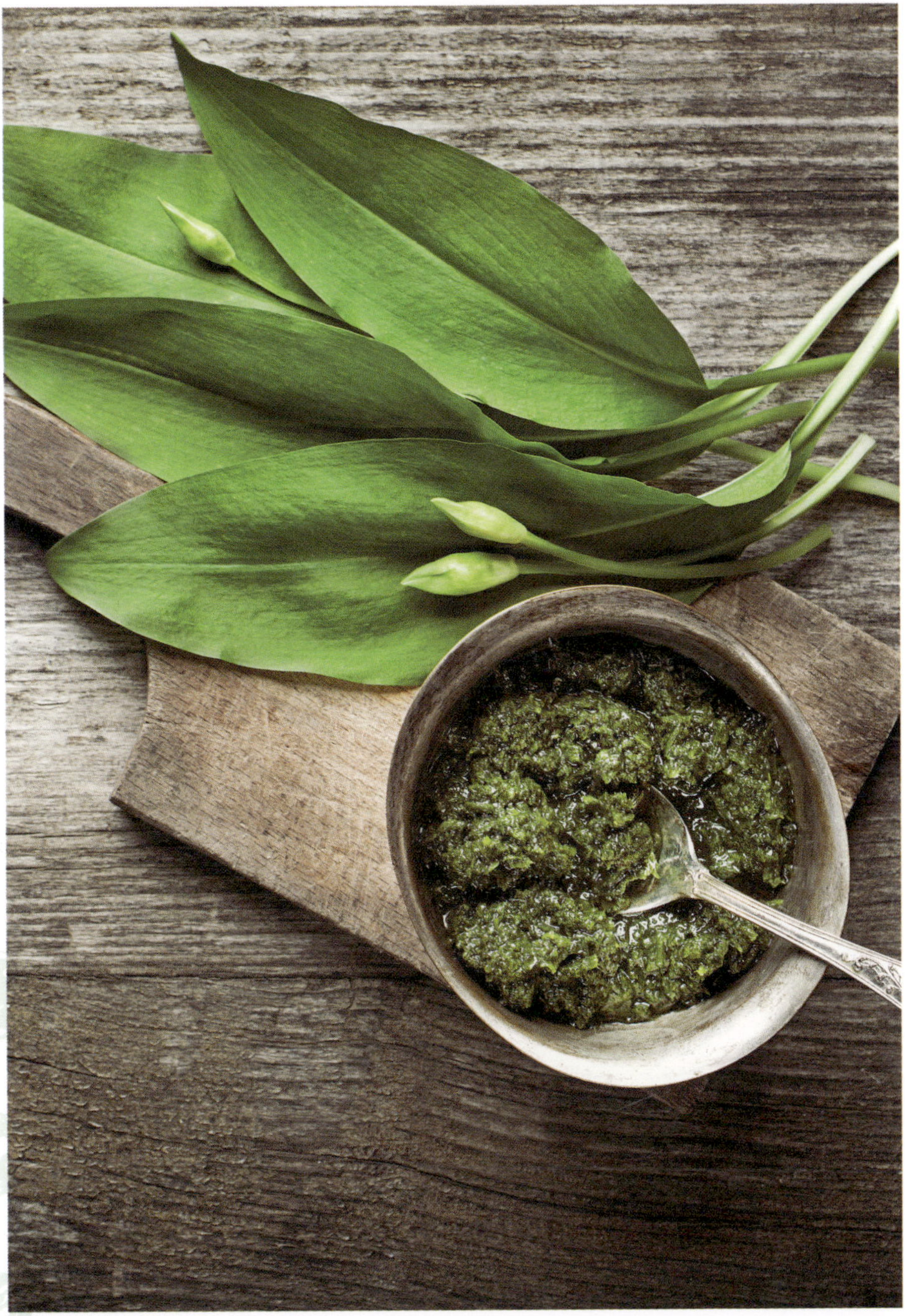

SEASONAL SLOW RECIPES

Embrace sustainable, seasonal and local foods with this selection of recipes.

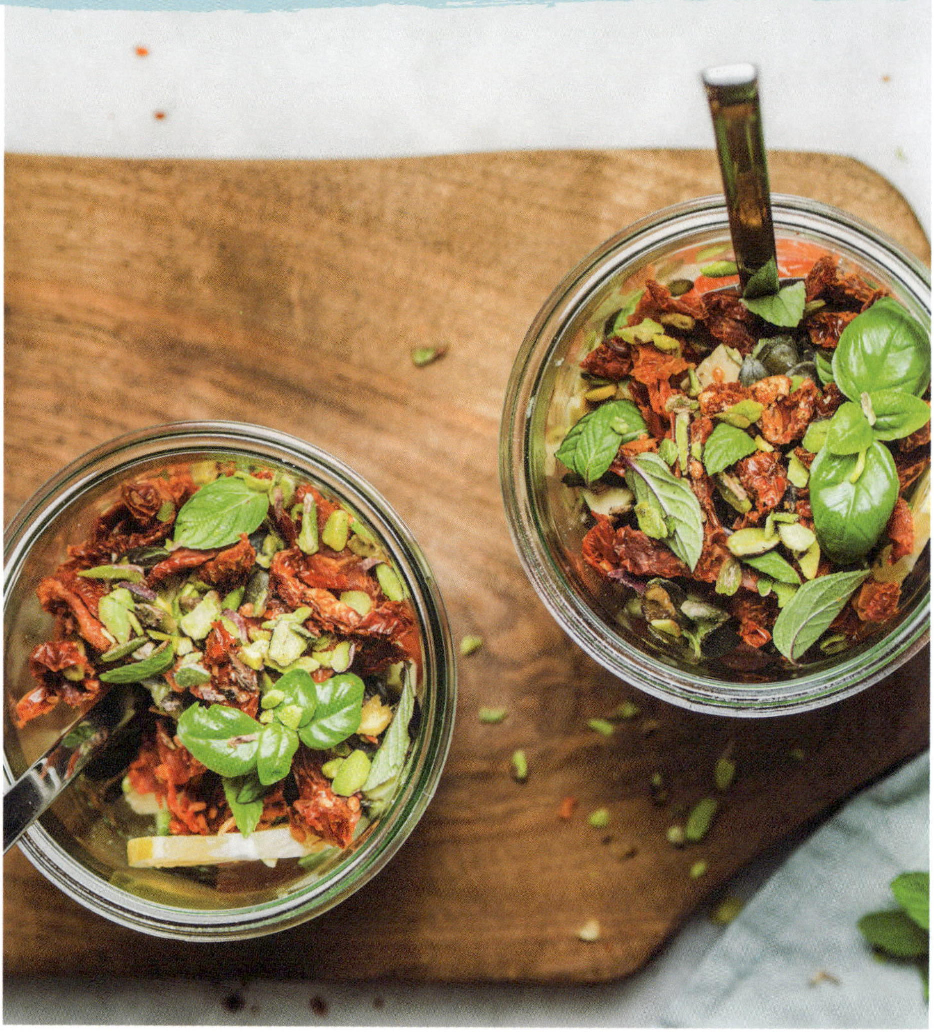

SPRING SALAD JAR

SERVES FOUR

Butterhead lettuces are floppy-leafed varieties available throughout the year. Winter-friendly varieties such as Arctic King or All Year Round will be harvested in spring and make great bases for zingy little jar-salads. The sweetness of the fresh spring peas contrasts well with the cut of the mustard seeds.

PREPARATION TIME:

20 minutes

COOKING TIME:

None

INGREDIENTS:

3 tbsp olive oil
1 tbsp lemon juice
1 tbsp cider vinegar
400 g (14 oz) peas
1 head butterhead lettuce
3 tsp coriander seeds
3 tsp mustard seeds
Handful baby basil leaves
Optional extras:
Sundried tomatoes
Chopped nuts and seeds, such as pistachio nuts and sunflower seeds
Mint leaves
Thinly sliced lemon pieces
Chilli flakes

METHOD

Whisk the oil, juice and vinegar together and pour into the base of four jars.

Boil the peas for 5 minutes then drain and cool. Add a layer to each of the jars.

Wash the lettuce, pat dry and tear into medium pieces. Add a layer to each jar.

Crush the coriander seeds, mix with the mustard seeds and add to each jar.

Finish with the baby basil leaves and toppings of your choice.

PAN-FRIED COD
WITH SUMMER POTATO JUMBLE

SERVES FOUR

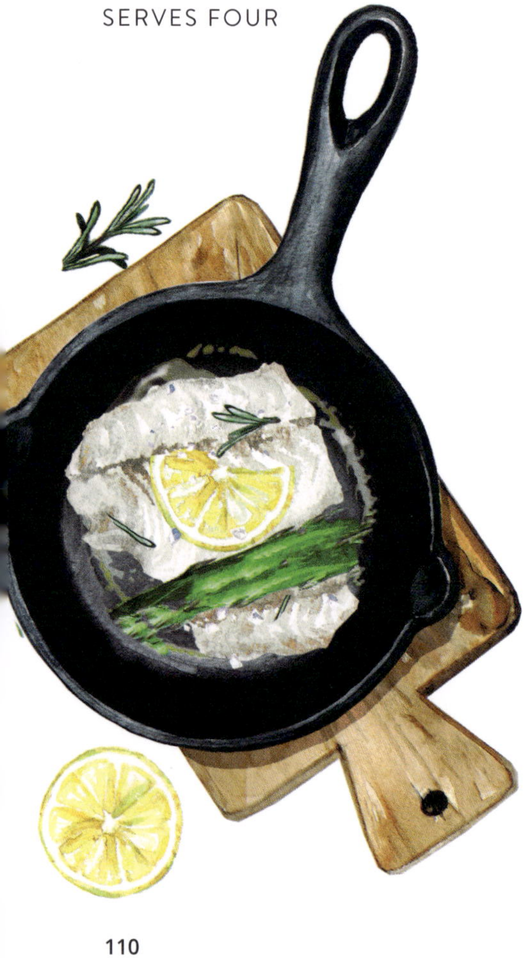

PREPARATION TIME:
12 hours, 10 minutes

COOKING TIME:
30 minutes

INGREDIENTS:

100 g (3½ oz) cherry tomatoes
Pinch salt, plus extra for seasoning
Pinch sugar
Glug olive oil, plus enough to cover a pan
2 tbsp plain flour
¼ tsp black pepper, plus extra for seasoning
¼ tsp paprika
2 tsp lemon zest
4 cod fillets*
500 g (17½ oz) new potatoes
Handful sage leaves
1 lemon
100 g (3½ oz) spinach leaves
Handful basil leaves
150 g (5¼ oz) pitted green and black olives
1 red chilli

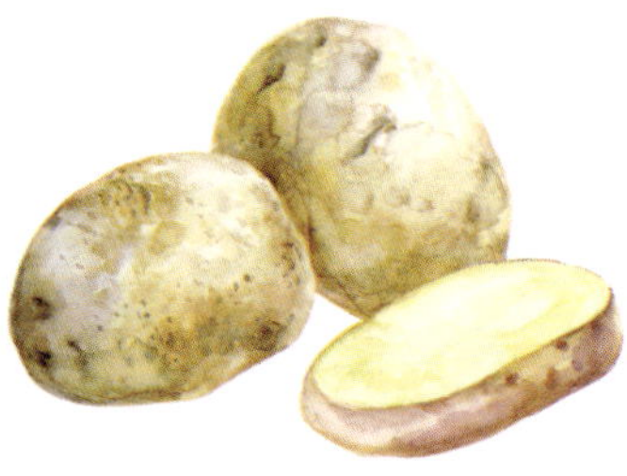

Summer is the season of abundance, and your dishes can overflow with taste and texture without trespassing into stodginess. By late August, the cherry tomatoes, olives and chillies will be ripe and ready to add their customary punch of flavour. Paired with lemon, earthy sage reminds the palate of its Mediterranean origins.

METHOD

Prepare the tomatoes the evening before you plan to make the dish. Preheat the oven to 200°C/400°F/Gas Mark 6. Slice in half and lay face up in an ovenproof dish. Sprinkle salt and sugar over them and then drizzle the oil. Put in the oven and turn off the heat. Remove from the oven the next morning or at least 8 hours later. The tomatoes should appear slightly shrivelled and will be intensely flavoured. Store in the fridge until you're ready to use them.

Mix the flour, a pinch of salt, pepper, paprika and lemon zest together. Dip your fish fillets in the mixture until coated. Put aside until you're ready to use them.

Cut the potatoes in half and boil until nearly soft, around 15 minutes. Drain and pat dry with kitchen roll.

Add enough olive oil to a deep pan so that the base is completely covered but not with any depth. Shallow fry the potatoes until golden brown on one side. Sprinkle in salt and pepper and then toss in the pan for around 10–15 minutes until completely cooked but not burned.

Remove potatoes from the pan and add olives and chilli. Cook for 5 minutes, keeping the ingredients moving.

Meanwhile, heat 2 tbsp olive oil in a separate pan, adding sage leaves a few at a time and frying for 20 seconds each. Remove the leaves and let them sit on kitchen roll.

With the heat on high, place the fish in the pan and fry until crispy, around 5 minutes. Cut the lemon into rounds and place on top. Cook for a further 3 minutes until the flesh is opaque.

Meanwhile, add the spinach, tomatoes and basil to the olives and chilli and warm through for 1–2 minutes. Return the potatoes to the pan and toss together.

Spoon the potato mixture onto the plate and add the fish on top. Garnish with the cooked sage leaves and serve with seasonal greens.

* Cook according to the catch of the day. If cod is not available at your local fishmonger, use haddock, pollock, black cod, striped bass, grouper or hake.

AUTUMN VEGETABLE PAELLA

SERVES FOUR

PREPARATION TIME:

10 minutes

COOKING TIME:

1 hour

INGREDIENTS:

2 small harlequin squash
2 tbsp olive oil
2 medium onions
4 cloves garlic
1 courgette
1 red pepper
1 yellow pepper
2 tomatoes
2 tsp paprika
½ tsp saffron
800 ml (27 fl oz) vegetable stock
400 g (14 oz) paella rice
1 bunch parsley
Handful cashew nuts

METHOD

Heat the oven to 180°C/350°F/Gas Mark 4 and roast the whole squash for an hour. Start cooking the paella 15 minutes after placing the squash in the oven.

Heat the oil. Finely chop the onions and garlic and add to the pan. Cook for 3 minutes until soft.

Dice the courgette and peppers and stir in. Cover and cook for a further 3 minutes.

Meanwhile, chop the tomatoes. Uncover the pan, make a well in the centre of the mix and add the tomatoes and paprika. Dissolve the saffron in the stock and add.

Stir the rice in gently and simmer until the liquid is absorbed and the rice is cooked. If the stock is absorbed and the rice still has bite, add more water.

A few minutes before the rice is done, stir in the parsley and the nuts. Remove the squash from the oven, cut in half and hollow out the stringy middle.

Add half a squash to each plate and heap the paella over it.

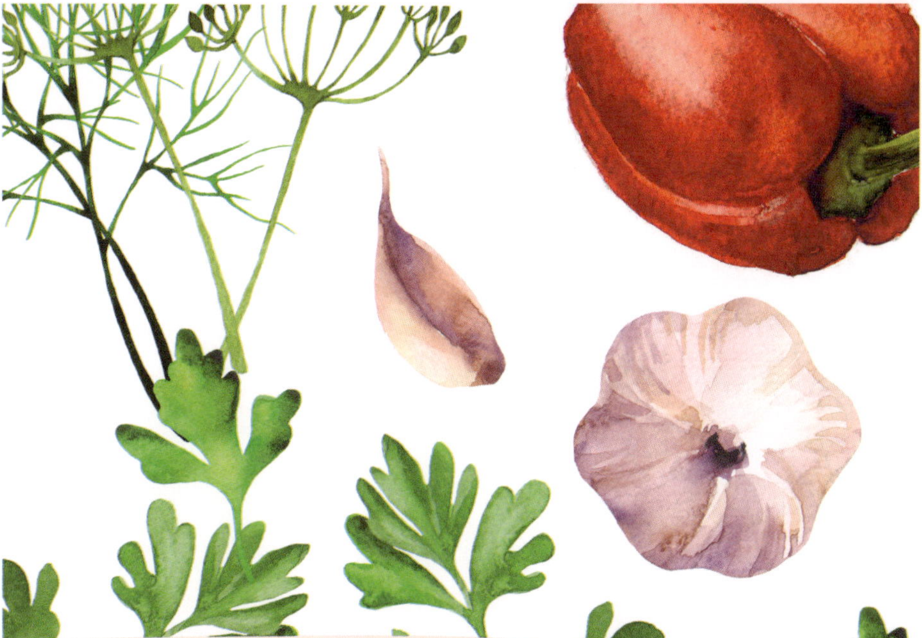

From the leaves on the trees to the crops in the field and garden, nature is set alight in autumn. The flecks of red, green and gold in this smoky paella certainly speak to this season of dwindling sunlight, although the sweet bursts of pepper remind us that we still have a handful of warm, blue-sky days yet to enjoy.

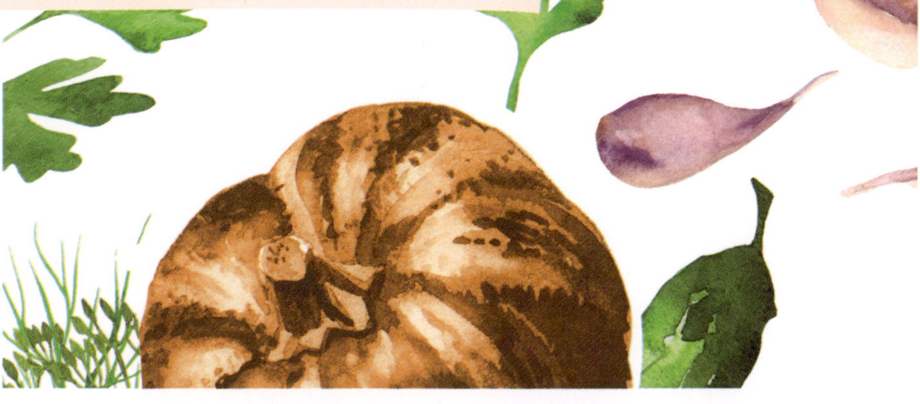

WINTER SLOW COOKER RIBOLLITA

SERVES SIX

PREPARATION TIME:
10 minutes

COOKING TIME:
8 hours, 45 minutes

INGREDIENTS:

- 2 medium onions
- 200 g (7 oz) carrots
- 300 g (10½ oz) celery
- 1 fennel bulb
- 4 cloves garlic
- 2 bay leaves
- 1 kg (2¼ lb) ham hock
- 400 g tin chopped tomatoes
- 3 sprigs fresh rosemary
- 1 tsp dried chilli flakes
- 2 litres (3½ pints) vegetable stock
- 350 g (12¼ oz) curly kale
- 400 g tin cannellini beans
- 250 g (8¾ oz) slightly stale country-style or sourdough bread
- 40 g (1½ oz) Parmesan cheese

METHOD

Chop one onion and the carrots finely, slice the celery and fennel thinly and quarter the remaining onion. Crush the garlic. Add these ingredients to the slow cooker with the bay leaves, ham hock, tin of tomatoes (undrained), rosemary, chilli and vegetable stock. Cook on low for 8 hours.

Remove the ham from the cooker and set aside to cool. Add the curly kale and cannellini beans. Cook on high until the kale is completely wilted.

When the ham is comfortable to touch, shred the meat from the bone. Don't use the fat, skin or bone. (You can make ham stock for the future if you have any spare onion, celery and carrot leftover. Chop them finely, combine with the bone and cover with water. Simmer on low for 40 minutes and strain.)

Add the meat back into the slow cooker and season to taste.

Tear the bread into chunks and add a handful to each bowl. Cover with the soup and grate the Parmesan over it.

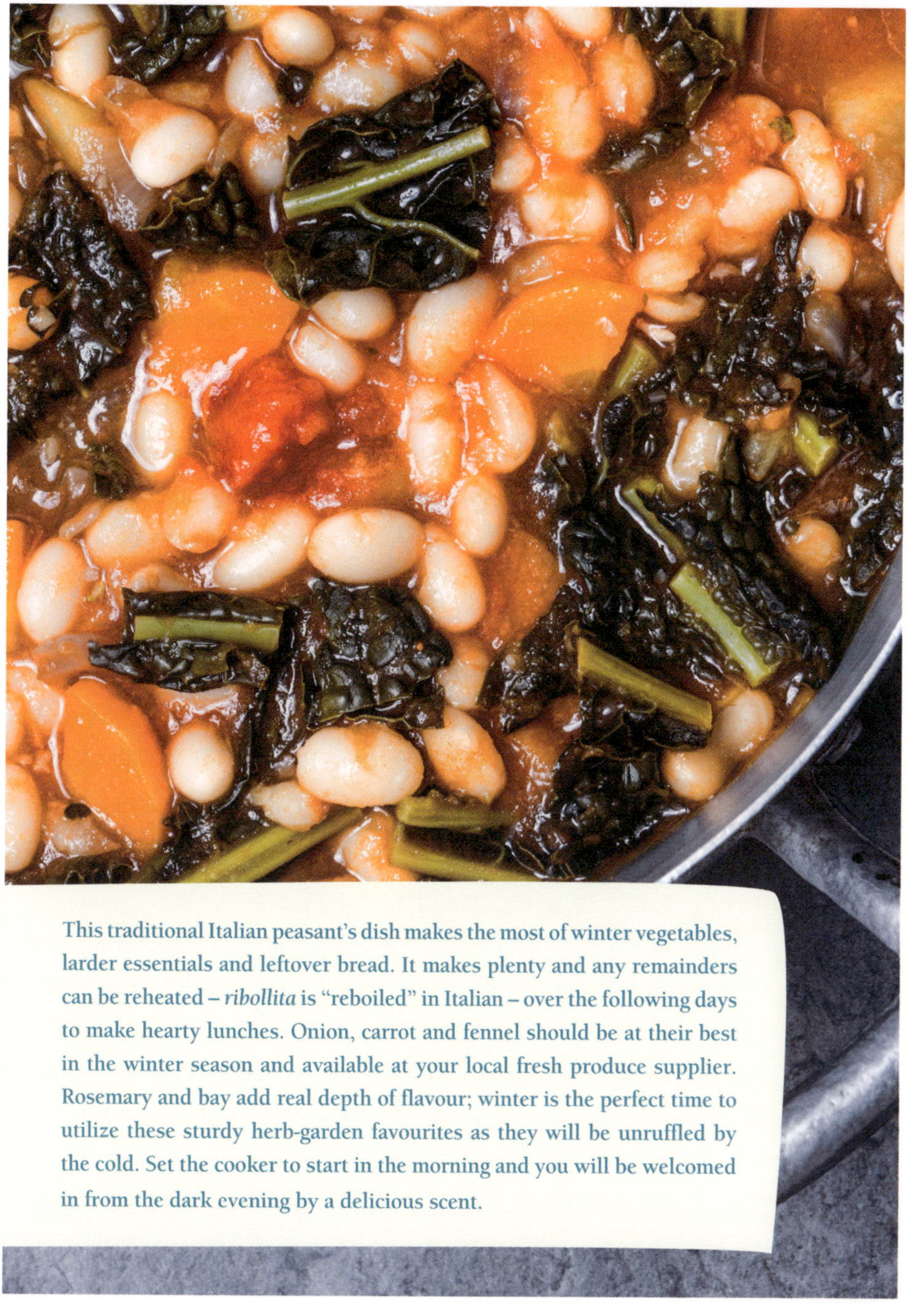

This traditional Italian peasant's dish makes the most of winter vegetables, larder essentials and leftover bread. It makes plenty and any remainders can be reheated – *ribollita* is "reboiled" in Italian – over the following days to make hearty lunches. Onion, carrot and fennel should be at their best in the winter season and available at your local fresh produce supplier. Rosemary and bay add real depth of flavour; winter is the perfect time to utilize these sturdy herb-garden favourites as they will be unruffled by the cold. Set the cooker to start in the morning and you will be welcomed in from the dark evening by a delicious scent.

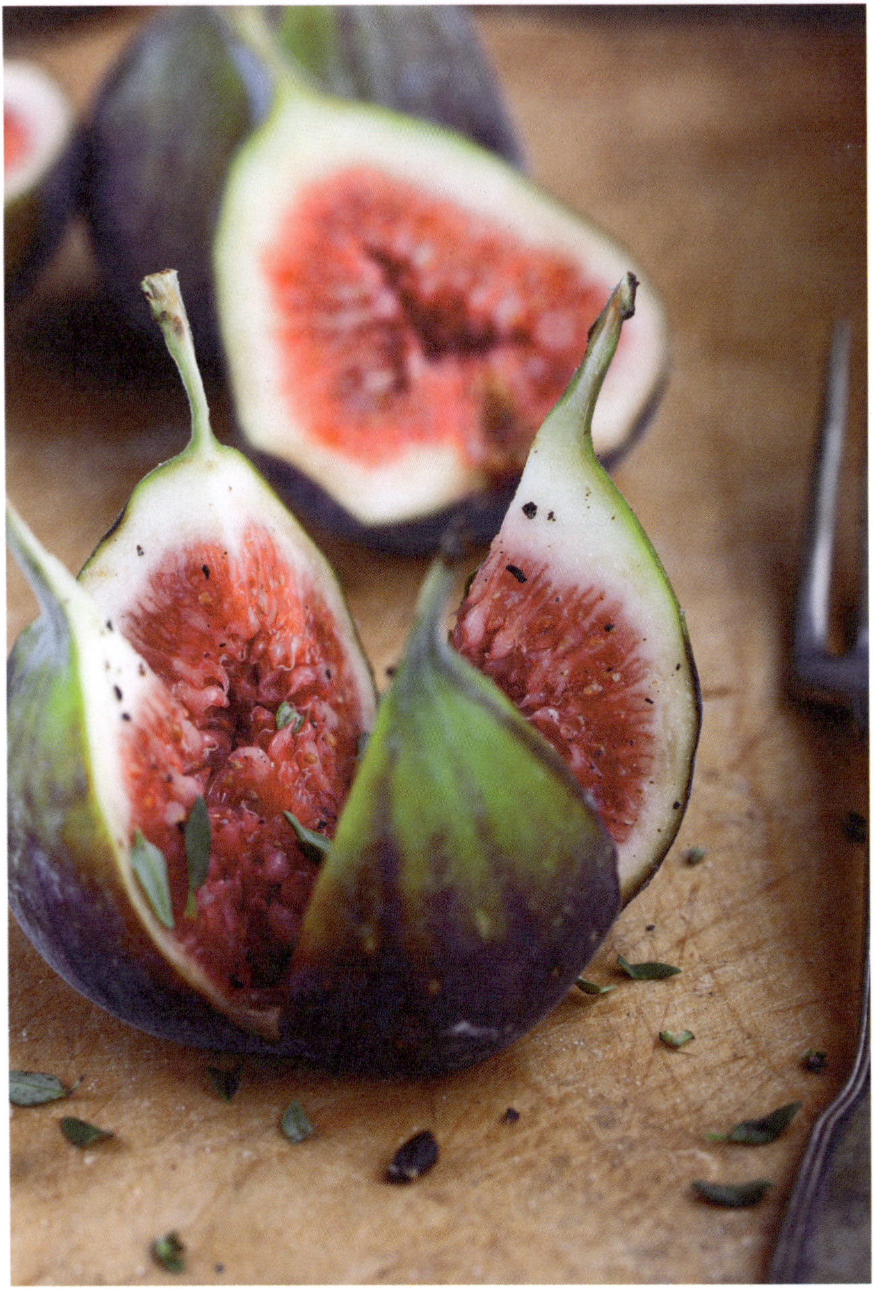

SLOW MOMENT

Tune in to your body to find out what it needs. If you are craving a sugary snack, stop and think about how you are feeling. People often self-soothe by eating sugary foods when they're feeling stressed. Be fully aware of this craving, as the awareness will lessen the desire. Maybe you don't need that chocolate bar after all.

SLOW WORK

This can be the trickiest area to overhaul when adopting a slow lifestyle. How can one possibly slow down and still maintain efficiency? Studies into time management by research groups such as the Centre for Time Use Research show that most people feel that they simply do not have enough time in the day to do everything they need to. Does this sound familiar? These same research groups have analyzed the leisure time of the modern European or American and found that, if anything, we have more leisure time than ever before. People, on average, spend no more time working now than in the past and, in fact, they spend more time with their families.

So why do we feel so rushed? Part of the reason may be that we can do so much with ease that it's making our lives harder! Technology has made it so that we can achieve many things in a short amount of time. Although that sounds great, it trips us up in two ways. Firstly, we seem to value the time spent doing a task as much as having completed the task itself. So although you've just ticked three items off your list in an hour, you barely feel as though you've achieved anything. Secondly, it's that multitasking can actually have a negative effect on your brain. Skipping between tasks quickly and with no breaks uses more energy than if you complete tasks one at a time and with some recharge time in-between. Not only that, but some studies show that multitasking can have the same effect on your brain as alcohol or marijuana, slowing your reaction times and your cognitive ability. Although you shouldn't entirely eschew the benefits of modern technology, be sure to build small breaks into your chores and exchange multitasking for single-tasking. This chapter offers practical ways to introduce a more comfortable rhythm into your work life.

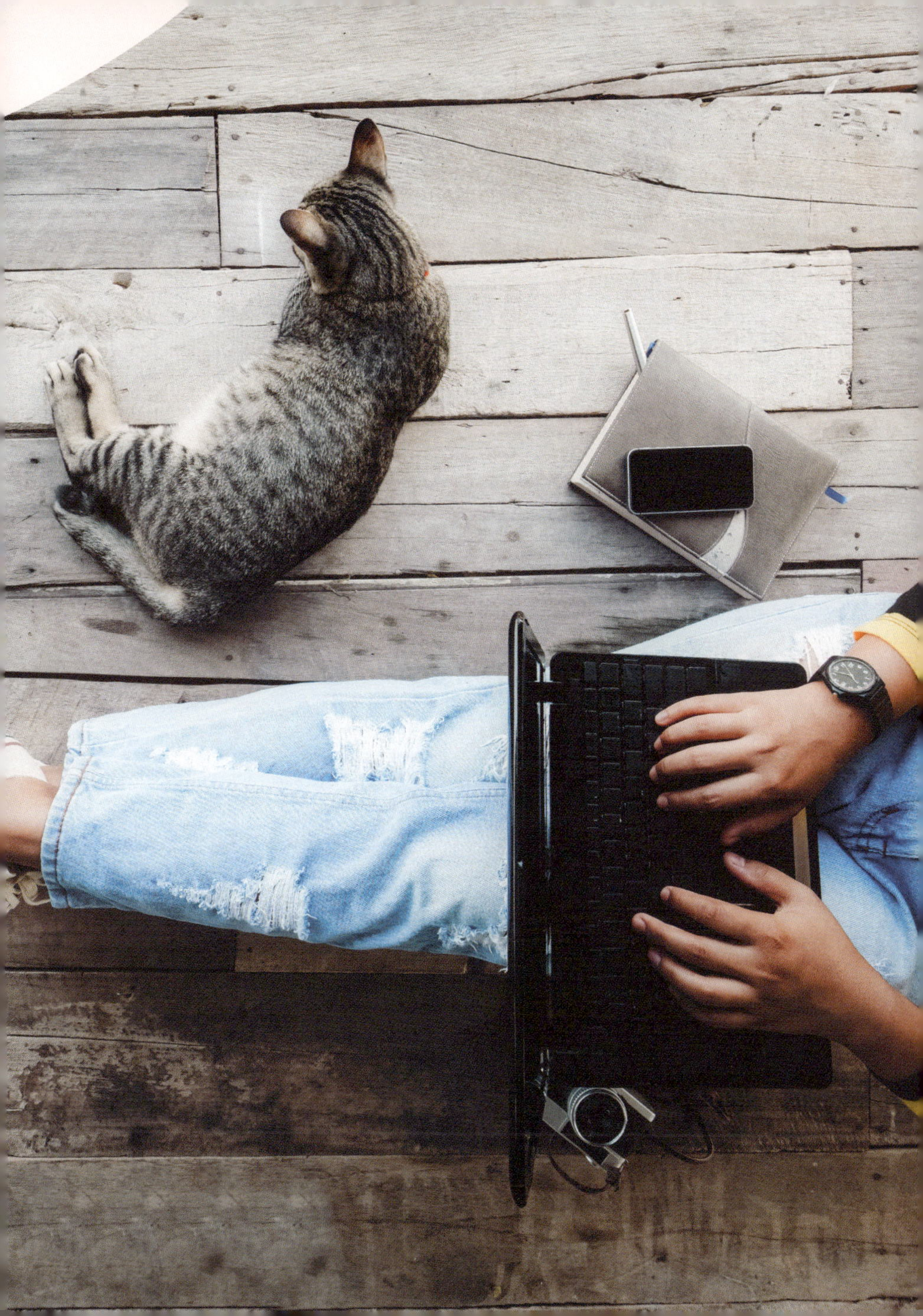

SLOW MOMENT

Geir Berthelsen, founder of The World Institute of Slowness (a think tank for adopting a slow lifestyle), recommends greater interaction in the workplace as an effective way to slow down and improve efficiency. Try smiling at people, being sincere, respecting opinions, showing interest in others, being considerate of others' feelings and being ready to help. Keep these ideas in mind when you're going about your daily tasks.

TO-DO LIST:

- [x] Don't overdo your to-do list
- [ ]
- [ ]
- [ ]
- [ ]
- [ ]
- [ ]
- [ ]
- [ ]
- [ ]

YOU CAN DO

ANYTHING

BUT NOT

EVERYTHING.

DAVID ALLEN

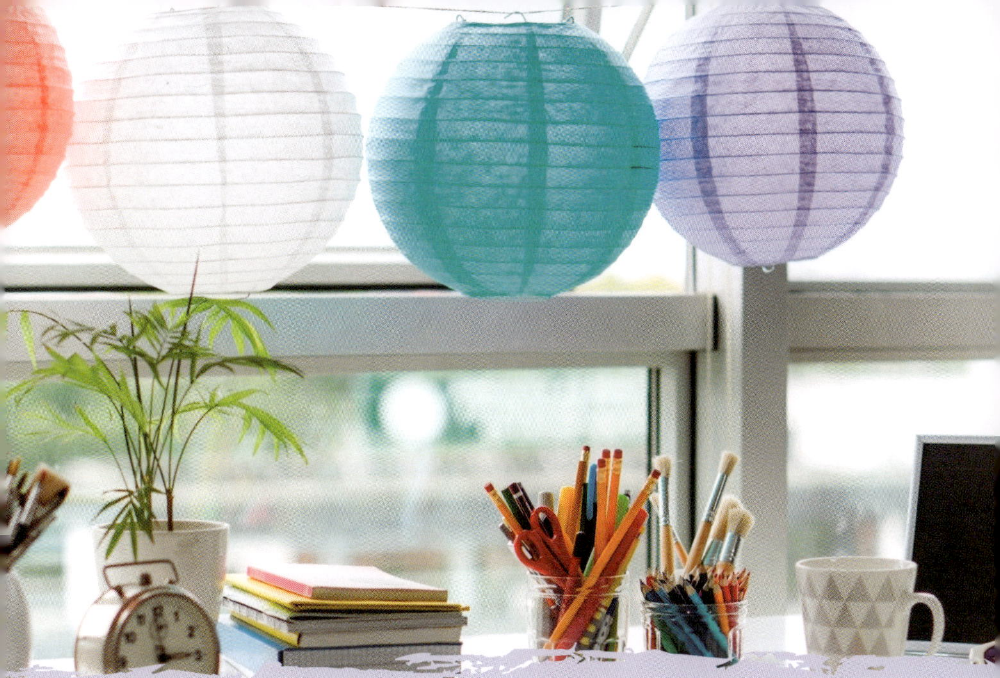

SINGLE-TASKING

Multitasking has become embedded as one of the key working principles in office life for promoting efficiency and productivity. Being perpetually busy has become the accepted norm, and not being busy is almost tantamount to failure. But common sense and research will tell you otherwise. We are most productive when focusing on one task at a time – it's how our brains work best. If you're juggling a number of jobs, then you will not have your full concentration on any of them. This scattered thinking leads to mistakes and a slowing down of productivity and competence levels. Multitasking is also less conducive to creative thinking, creates elevated levels of cortisol that impair cognitive function, and it's downright stressful having to keep track of each task as you jump between them, so stop! The next time you have a number of tasks bustling for attention, be kind to yourself and try single-tasking instead, and experience the satisfaction of completing a single task to the best of your ability. Try out the prompts on the following page to become a super single-tasker.

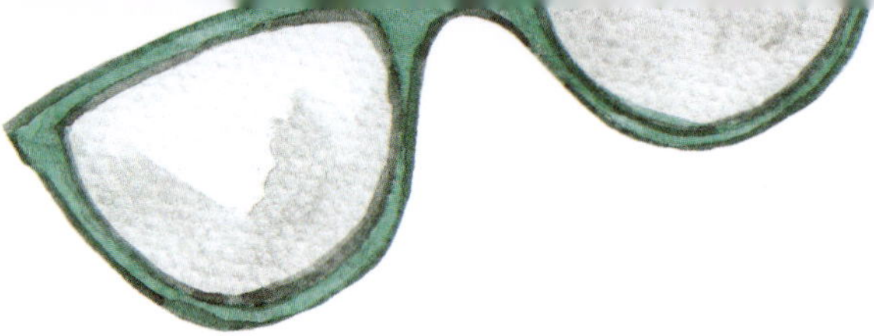

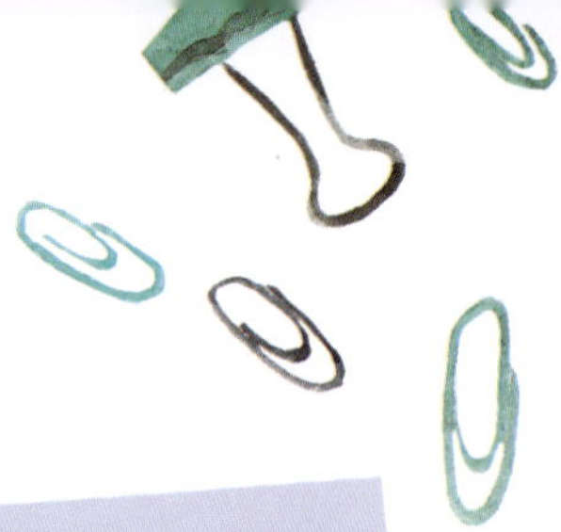

Try out these prompts to become a super single-tasker.

Cut out distractions

Do you need to have your emails and web browser open or an instant messenger minimized in the corner of your screen while you're writing a report? Close all applications that distract you from your job. If you have the luxury of your own office, close the door, or if you're in an open-plan office, let your colleagues know to keep the banter down and that you will not be answering emails. Then there are other distractions, the ones inside your head – thoughts and worries lining up, jostling for attention. We each have unique tendencies or thoughts that pull us away from the task at hand. Start paying attention to your thoughts and jot down the ones that distract you most often. Do you have a tendency to dwell on the past or the future? Are you consumed with thoughts of guilt, fear or worry? Do you ruminate on achieving perfection? Writing these tendencies down can help you become more mindful about what is going on in your head when you stray from the present moment and your job.

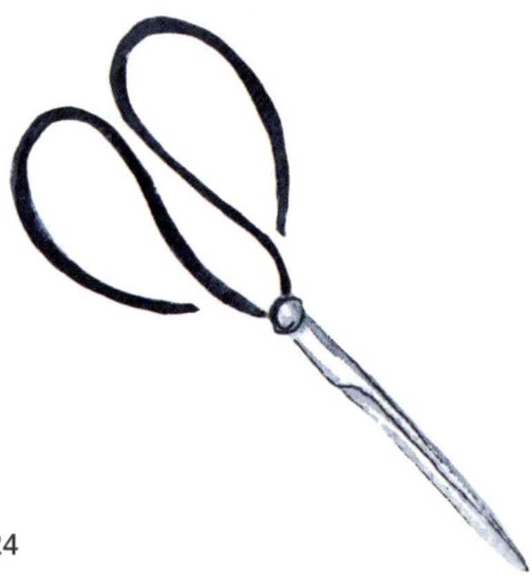

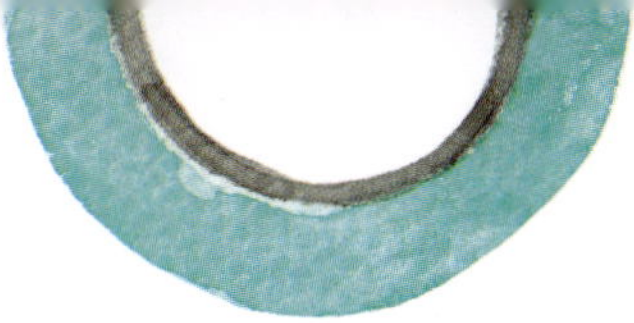

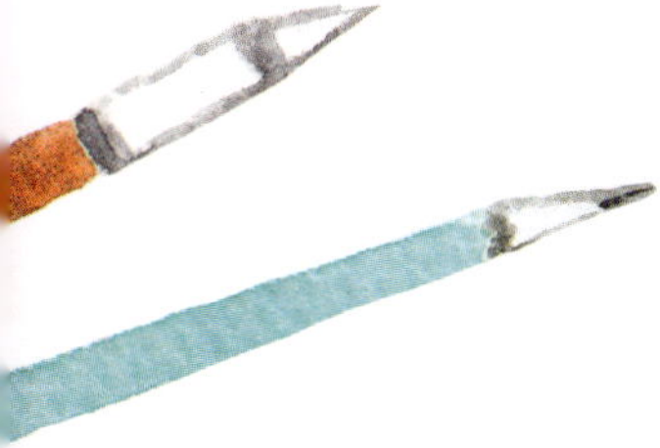

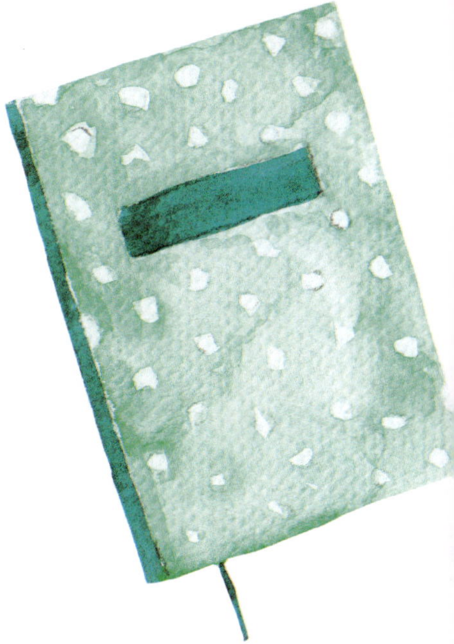

Learn your work patterns

We're all different in terms of productivity levels and focus, but learning when you are at your most productive is very useful for maximizing your efficiency. Whether you're a morning or afternoon person in terms of concentration levels, capitalize on this and focus on the jobs that require sustained and complex thought at the right time. Use the times when you're not feeling as focused for quick-win jobs, such as answering emails and organizing your schedule.

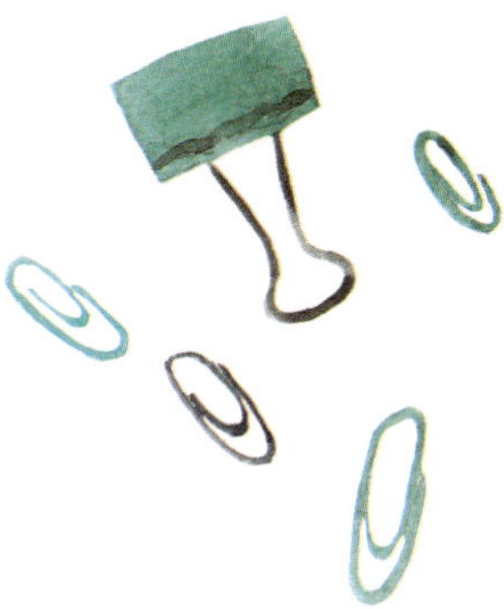

Decide what's most important

It can be tricky to work out what's most important, or what should be done first. To help with this, limit yourself to three or four urgent tasks, consider which ones will have the most impact and begin with those, but single-task them. Try not to make this a morning job, as this can elevate stress levels before the working day has even begun. Make this an end-of-day job, so you're prepared for the morning and can focus as soon as you reach your workplace.

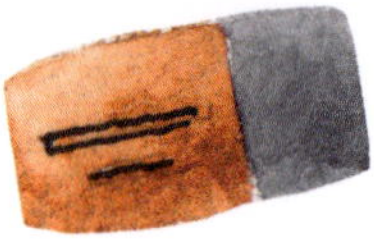

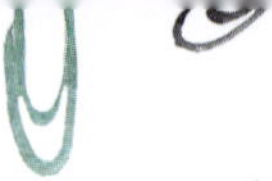

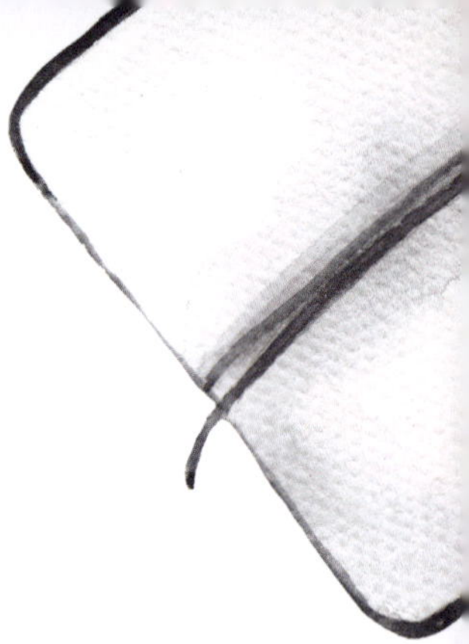

Maintaining focus

Multitasking can be a tough discipline to extract yourself from. If you struggle to stay focused on one job, get yourself a timer – preferably one that doesn't tick noisily – and begin by giving yourself 15 minutes to spend on a job without distraction. Gradually increase the amount over time, working up to longer periods of an hour or so.

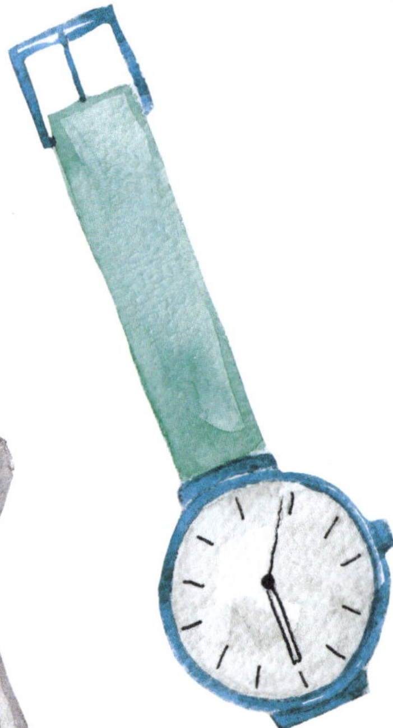

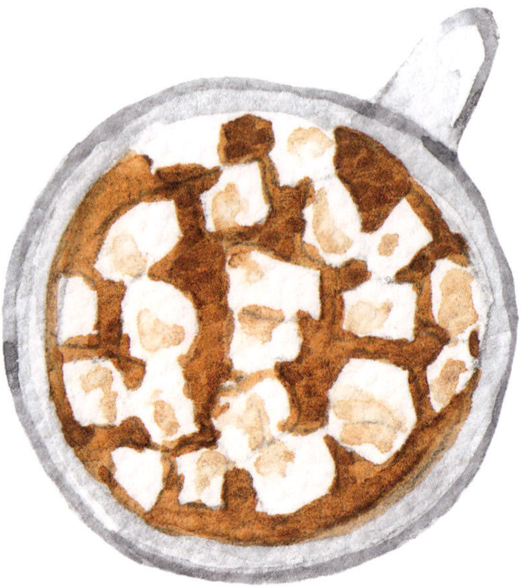

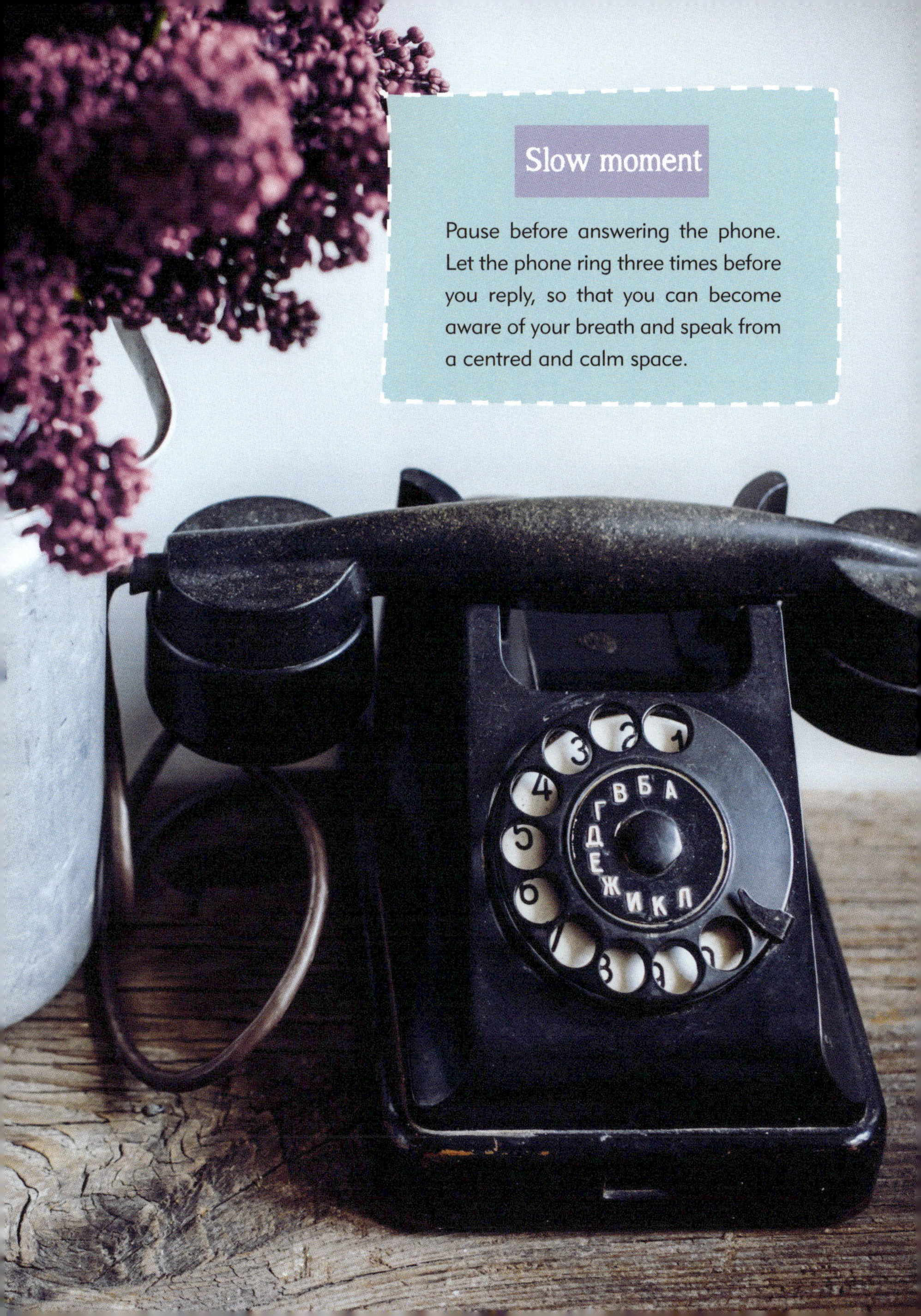

Slow moment

Pause before answering the phone. Let the phone ring three times before you reply, so that you can become aware of your breath and speak from a centred and calm space.

Start a bullet journal

These are a brilliantly low-tech way to organize your life, and it's surprisingly simple. You may wonder if reverting to paper from a digital organizer is taking an ill-advised step backwards, but analogue is more compliant with the way your brain works. A paper journal, as opposed to a digital one, engages our thought processes and helps us to absorb information more easily. A bullet journal starts life as a blank book. These are the key components ⇨

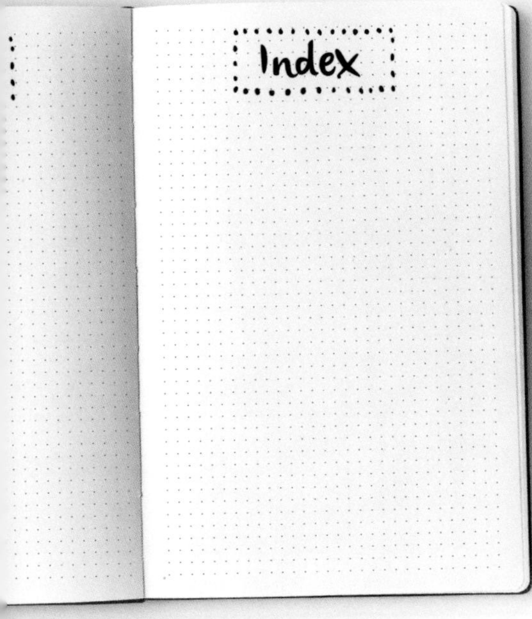

Index

This appears at the beginning of your journal and contains page titles and page numbers.

Future log

Store all future appointments, red-letter days and events here, until it's time to add the month in which they occur.

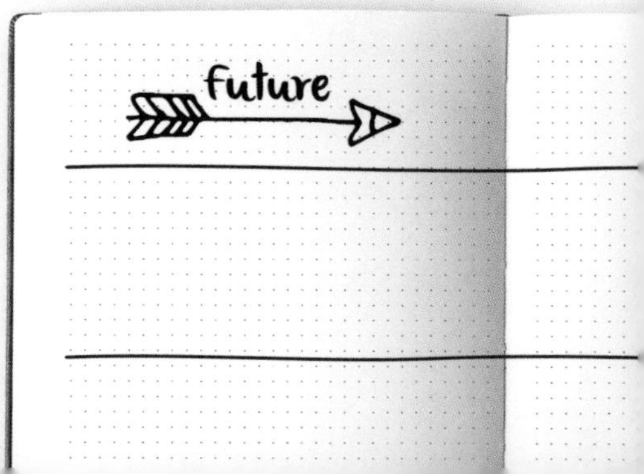

Monthly log

This shows the whole month on one page, what's due to happen on particular days, tasks to complete, and so on.

Daily log

Outline the tasks and appointments for each day, but remember to record special moments too – everything is of equal importance.

Create a key of symbols to apply to different levels or types of task to keep track of them. For example: draw a circle beside a task, then fill in the circle when it has been completed; a square for appointments, which is filled in when the appointment has happened; a star for very important tasks, and so on.

Once you are familiarized with the basics, you can personalize it further to your needs. For example: write down meal plans in your monthly log, then note down a shopping list at the start of each week in a weekly log; track goals – this could be exercise, writing, job applications – whatever is important to you to help you stay motivated; cleaning rota; birthday gift list; assignments and work deadlines.

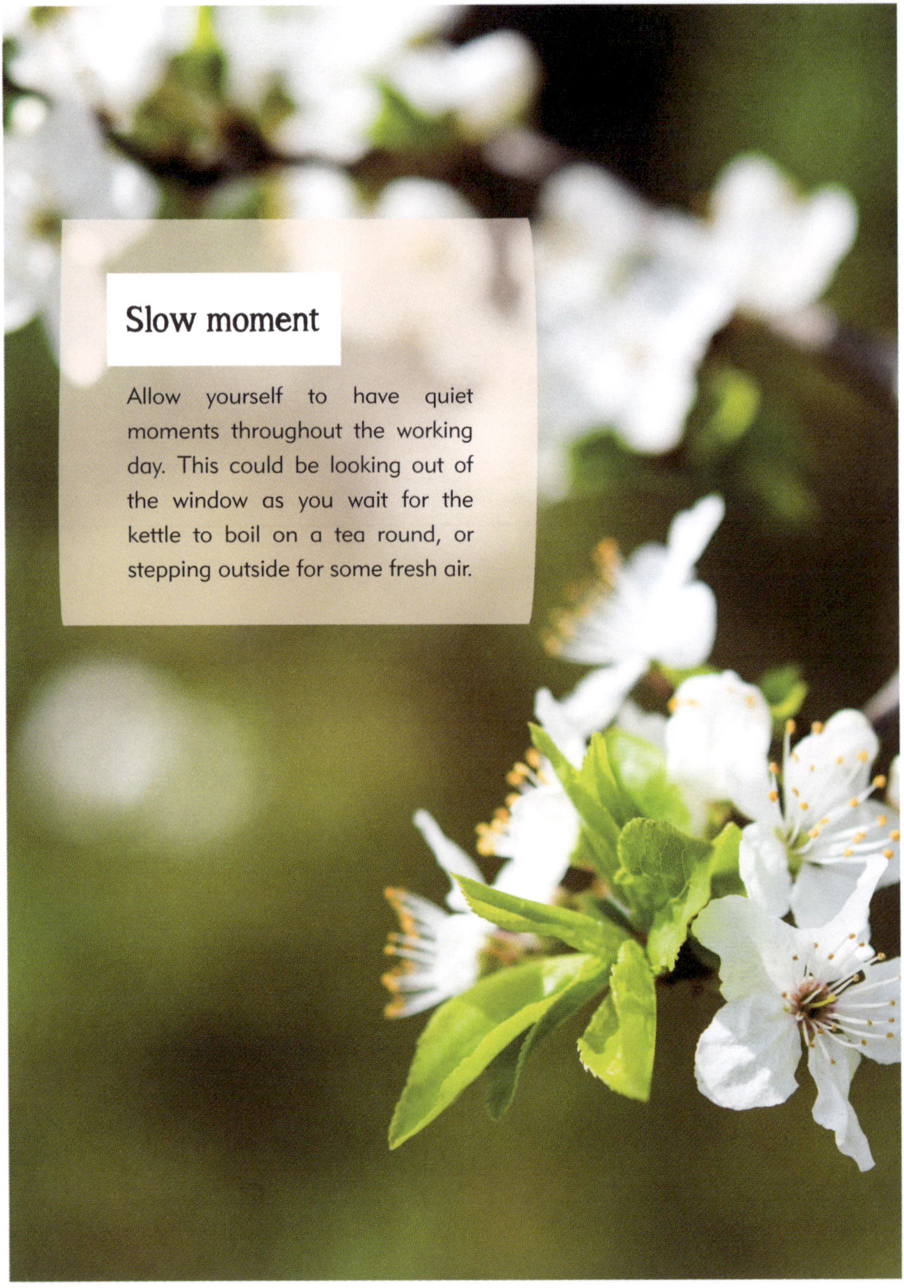

Slow moment

Allow yourself to have quiet moments throughout the working day. This could be looking out of the window as you wait for the kettle to boil on a tea round, or stepping outside for some fresh air.

STOP
a moment,
cease your work,
look
around
you.

LEO TOLSTOY

PAUSE

It's what gives you your power.

SLOW NATURE

When was the last time you turned off your gadgets, buttoned up your jacket and immersed yourself in nature? Spending time outdoors is the ideal way to reset and recharge, as you allow your mind to tick unhurried and notice the small details. Here are some ideas for enjoying the slow, simple pleasures of an outdoor lifestyle.

Don't hurry,
don't worry.
And be sure
to smell the
flowers along
the way.

WALTER HAGEN

TAKE A
FOREST BATH

Listening to the sound of the trees rustling and swaying, the satisfying crunch of autumn leaves underfoot, the glow of green leaves in summer, the call of a cuckoo – there are many simple pleasures to be enjoyed when spending time in the woods. The Japanese have a special term for it: forest bathing, which means being in the presence of trees. Forest bathing became part of the public health programme in Japan in the 1980s as research has proven that it has numerous benefits: it lowers heart rate and blood pressure, reduces stress hormone production, boosts the immune system and improves overall feelings of well-being.

Further research has shown that children who spend time in natural environments "perform better in reading, mathematics, science and social studies", and 80 per cent of the UK's happiest people say they have a connection with nature.

The forest is a therapeutic landscape, one that can be enjoyed without the need to accomplish anything – steps, for example – and everyone can reap the rewards.

So try a forest bath sometime! But if that's not enough of an incentive to get you, your family or your friends reaching for their coat and wellies, try out a few ideas in this book or let them spark ideas of your own – try building a den, go on a bug hunt or simply see how many different coloured and shaped leaves you can pick up off the forest floor. It's cheap, fun and healthy.

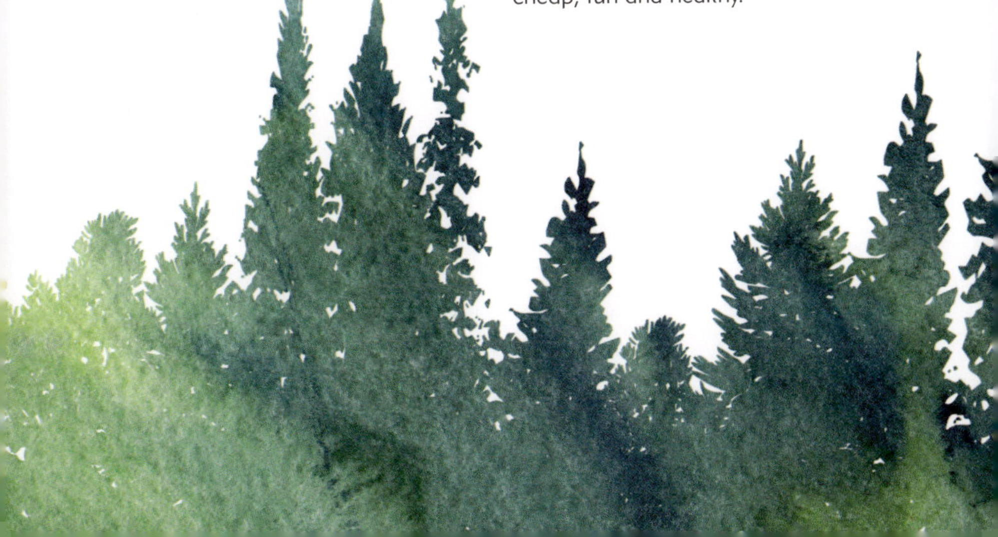

TIPS FOR SLOW RITUALS IN NATURE

Put out a bird feeder and watch garden birds flock to it

Enjoy the rain on your face

Stand at the top of a hill and take in the panorama, watch the shadows of clouds skim the landscape

Notice the silence

Jump in puddles

Lie on the grass and look up

Pick up stones on the beach and notice their textures

Wade into the sea and feel the draw of the tide

Match your breathing to the ebb and flow of the waves

Roll down a hill

Listen to the sounds around you: the wind, birdsong, running water, animal calls

Wade in a shallow stream

Watch fish swimming with the current

Wait for the stormiest weather, wrap up and enjoy the power of nature

Take off your socks and shoes and walk barefoot

Look for flowers, but don't pick them

Count the seconds between thunderclaps

Find a tree and sit beneath it – look up at the sunlight illuminating the leaves

Climb a tree, balance on a felled trunk, or simply wrap your arms around a tree and feel the texture of the bark on your face

Forage for sweet chestnuts, blackberries, sloes or whatever is in season

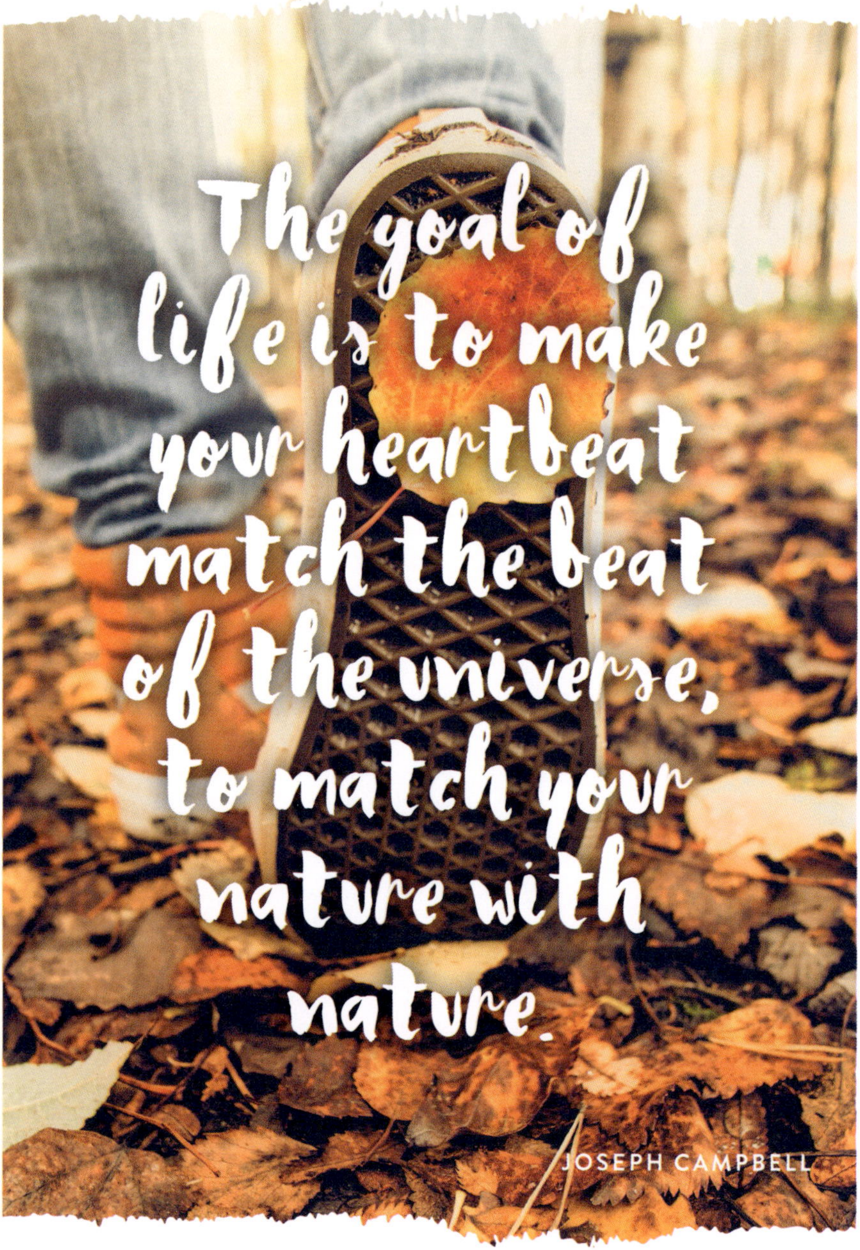
The goal of life is to make your heartbeat match the beat of the universe, to match your nature with nature.
JOSEPH CAMPBELL

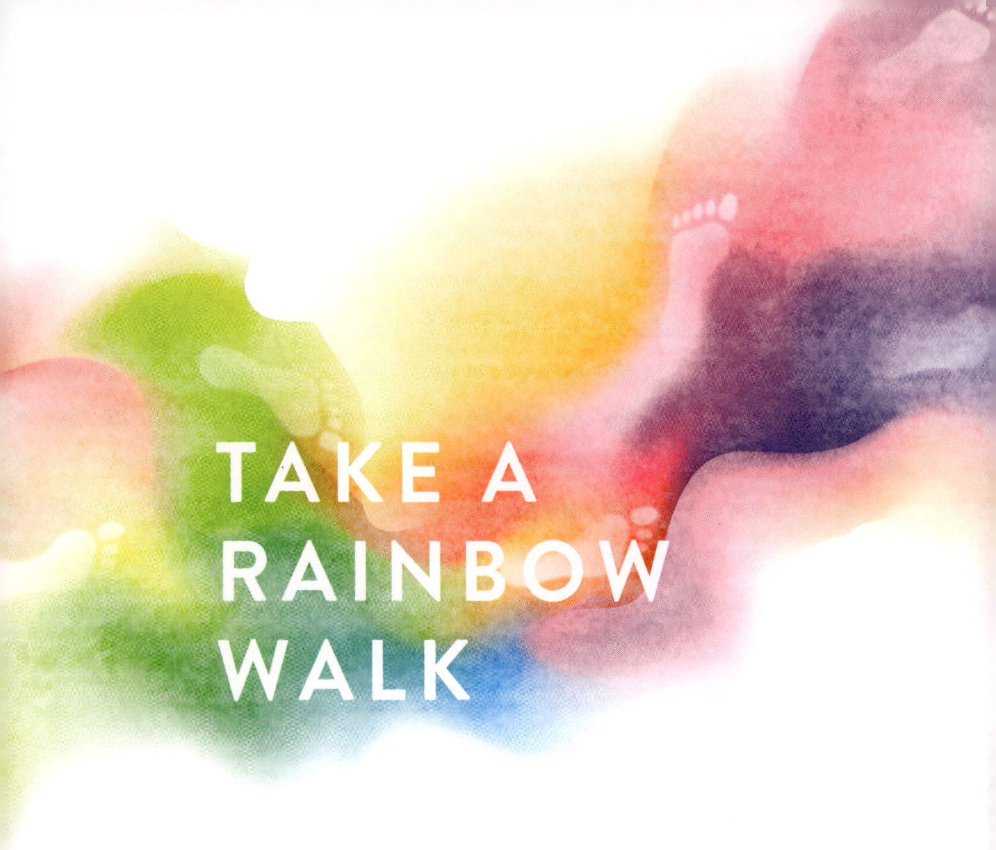

TAKE A RAINBOW WALK

This is a simple mindfulness exercise, which can be enjoyed at any time of year and helps you to remain present and notice your surroundings. It's also a fun game to play if you have company. The premise is simple – go for a walk and look for something red, then orange, then yellow, green, blue, indigo and violet. Then start again and repeat the rainbow until you have finished your walk.

TO BE BY THE SEA

Take a slow amble by the sea, away from traffic noise and people, and enjoy the sound of the waves, like slow breaths in and out. Look out to sea, a view with minimal distractions, and feel calm descend and stresses float away. Studies show that being in or around water – a quiet blue space – allows your brain to take a meditative break due to the limited levels of stimuli. The minerals and negative ions in sea air have been shown to be good for mental well-being by improving the flow of oxygen in our brains as well as balancing serotonin levels. If you don't live near the sea, find your own space close to home, which could be a river, reservoir or lake, and experience the positive effects to your well-being by being close to water.

SLOW MOMENT

If you're landlocked and in need of instant calm, take a restorative shower. It has a similar effect to being by the sea as it erases much of the stimulation that crowds your senses, allowing your brain to arrive at a mindful state. Showering also produces the same negative ions as sea air that help you to feel balanced and energized.

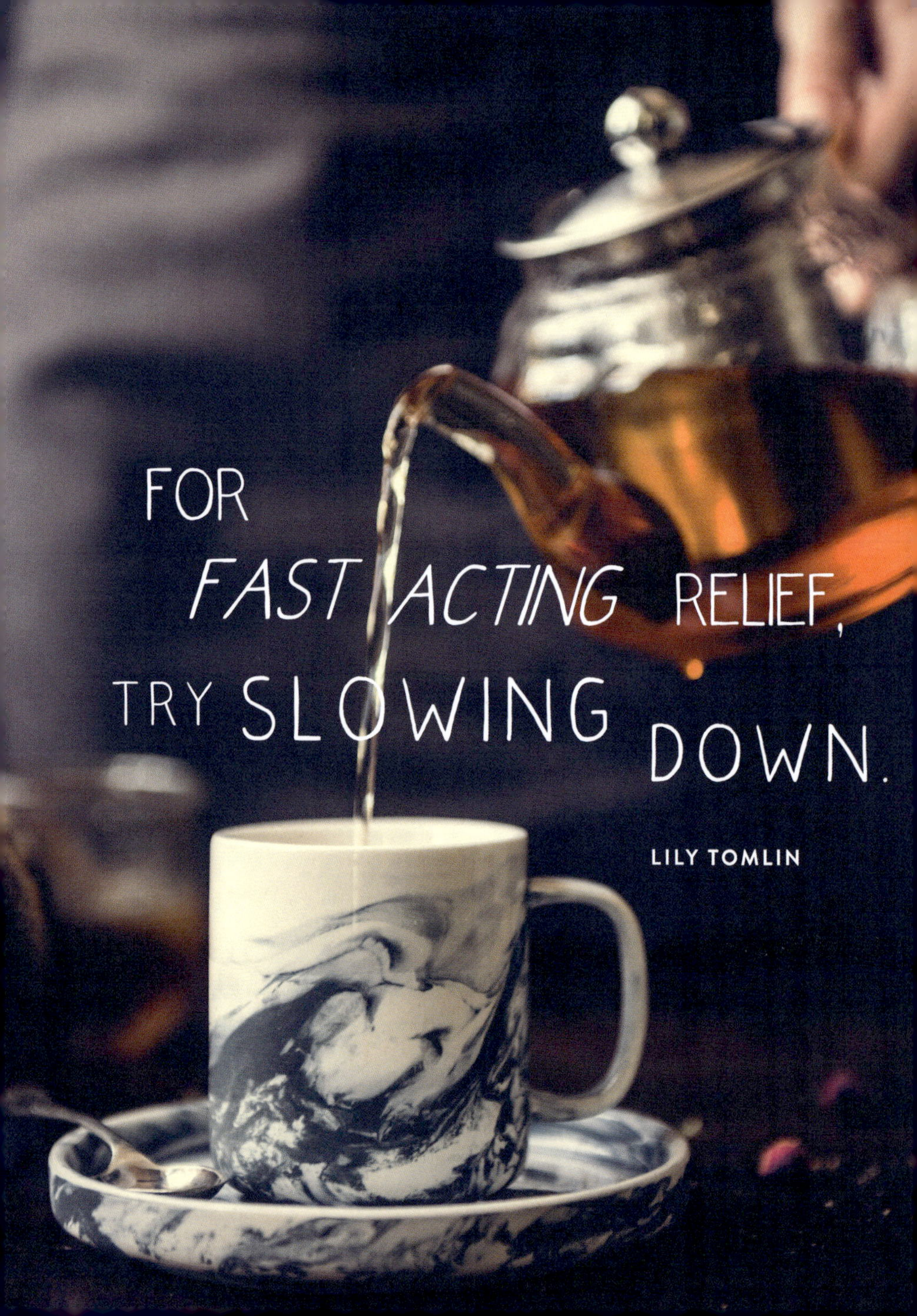
FOR
FAST ACTING RELIEF,
TRY SLOWING DOWN.
LILY TOMLIN

CONCLUSION

The constant switched-on nature of the modern world can be difficult to extract yourself from, but hopefully this book has offered you some practical solutions and processes to help you take a step back and assess how you can adopt a slow and more fulfilling lifestyle. Letting go of the compulsion to do all things, be all things and acquire material things can be liberating as well as hugely beneficial to your health and well-being. Simply nurture all that you are passionate about – health, happiness, relationships, work – and don't feel guilty about discarding the rest. Instead, enjoy the many benefits of a slower and more comfortable pace of life.

FURTHER RESOURCES

BULLET JOURNAL TUTORIALS

WWW.BULLETJOURNAL.COM

Ideas for creating a bullet journal.

WWW.LITTLECOFFEEFOX.COM

A beginner's guide to bullet journalling.

MINDFULNESS

WWW.MINDFUL.ORG/MEDITATION/MINDFULNESS-GETTING-STARTED

An organization with the mission to encourage the practice of mindfulness.

SLEEP

WWW.BRAIN.FM

Designed to send your mind into sleep mode with relaxing music (also available as an app).

WWW.RAINYMOOD.COM

Encourages you to relax by playing various sounds of rain on a loop (also available as an app).

SUDOKU AND PUZZLE

WWW.BRAIN-GAMES.CO.UK

Website containing many different games to keep your brain ticking.

WWW.JIGSAWPLANET.COM

An online way to solve your own jigsaw puzzles.

WWW.SUDOKU.COM

A fun and easy-to-use Sudoku website.

SUSTAINABLE LIFESTYLE

WWW.FRIENDS OFTHEEARTH.UK

An organization committed to leading a sustainable life and looking after the world we inhabit.

WWW.ILOVEFREEGLE.ORG

A volunteer organization promoting sustainable waste management practices.

WWW.RECYCLENOW.COM

England's government-funded national recycling campaign.

WWW.THEGREENAGE.CO.UK

The UK's main energy saving portal, advising people on how to make their businesses and homes as efficient as possible.

THE WORLD INSTITUTE OF SLOWNESS

WWW.THEWORLDINSTI-TUTEOFSLOWNESS.COM

A think tank promoting tackling organizational problems through slow thinking.

YOGA

WWW.BWY.ORG.UK

Website for The British Wheel of Yoga, which aims to increase people's knowledge and understanding of yoga across the country.

SLOW RECIPE BLOGS

WWW.RACHELKHOO.COM/ FOOD/SLOW-FOOD-RECIPES

Rachel's blog contains different slow food recipes for lunch and dinner, aimed to get back to the basics.

SLOW NOTES

Use these pages to jot down your own slow living ideas, recipes and memories.

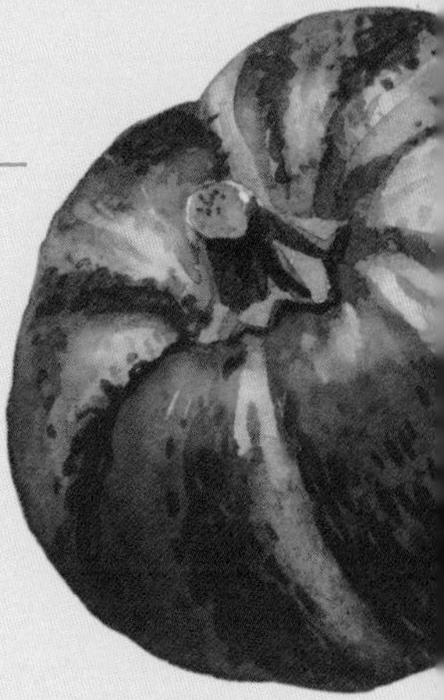

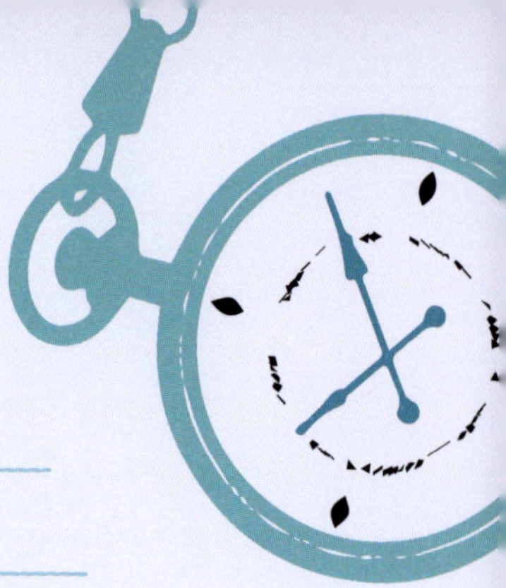

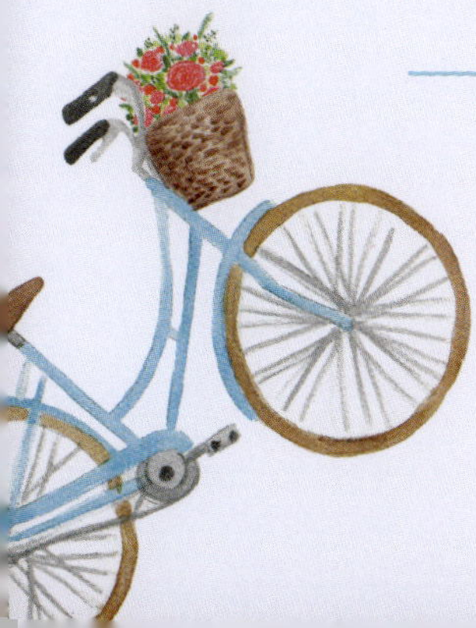

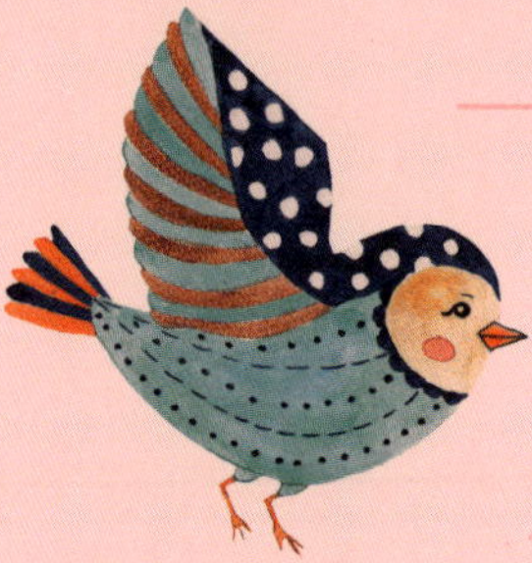

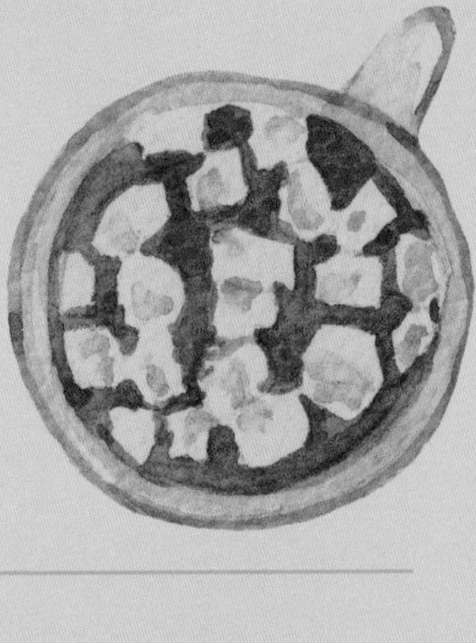

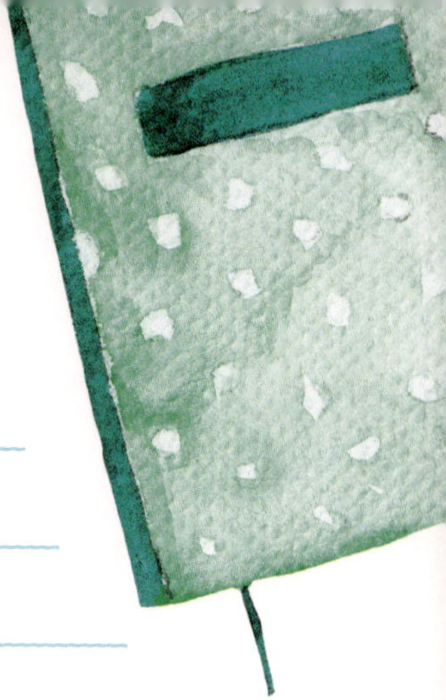

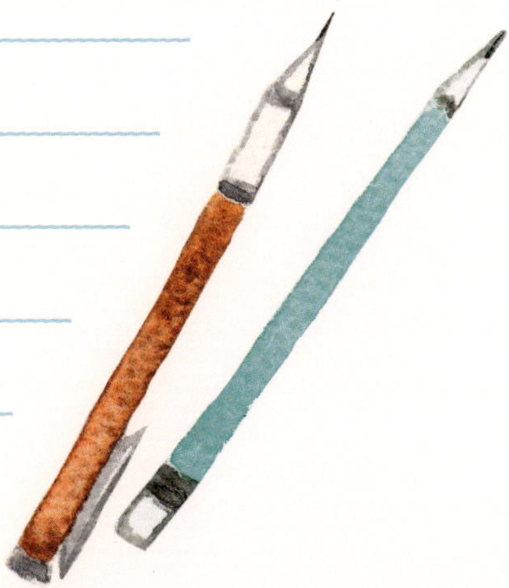

IMAGE CREDITS

pp.4–5 © watercolor 15/Shutterstock.com

pp.7, 146 © Rawpixel.com/Shutterstock.com

pp.8–9 background © arigato/Shutterstock.com; image © Siberica/Shutterstock.com

pp.10–11, 12–13 © Bogdan Sonjachnyj/Shutterstock.com

p.15 © mimagephotography/Shutterstock.com

pp.16–17 © Ivan Zhurba/Shutterstock.com

pp.18, 127, 132 © Daria Minaeva/Shutterstock.com

p.19 © 578foot/Shutterstock.com

p.20 ball of yarn © Le Chernina/Shutterstock.com

pp.22–23 © fototrips/Shutterstock.com

pp.24–25 © knahthra/Shutterstock.com

p.26 © Zikatuha /Shutterstock.com

p.27 © white snow/Shutterstock.com

pp.28–29, 94–95 © Yulia Grigoryeva/Shutterstock.com

pp.30, 31, 32, 33, 35 © Baleika Tamara/Shutterstock.com

p.34 © Babkina Svetlana/Shutterstock.com

p.36 © Khramtceva Mariya/Shutterstock.com

p.37 © Magnia/Shutterstock.com

pp.38–39 © ismailereny/Shutterstock.com

pp.40–41 © tsaplia/Shutterstock.com

pp.42–43 © Natalia Yankelevich/Shutterstock.com

pp.44–45 © Floral Deco/Shutterstock.com

p.46 © skyNext/Shutterstock.com

p.47 © exopixel/Shutterstock.com

pp.48, 49 © Lazerko A/Shutterstock.com

p.50 © matrioshka/Shutterstock.com

pp.52–53 © suns07butterfly/Shutterstock.com

pp.54, 56 © Ksusha Dusmikeeva/Shutterstock.com

p.55 © Andrekart Photography/Shutterstock.com

pp.56 (clock), 88–89 (clocks), 121, 160 © Tom Devonald

pp.58–59 © imnoom/Shutterstock.com

pp.60–61 © Angie Makes/Shutterstock.com

pp.62–63, 120, 124–125, 126, 152, 158, 159 © Elizaveta Ruzanova/Shutterstock.com

p.65 © Maria Savenko/Shutterstock.com

pp.66–67 © Uximetc pavel/Shutterstock.com

p.71 © Tayssa Marques/Shutterstock.com

pp.72–73 © Andrekart Photography/Shutterstock.com

p.74 © Zamurovic Photography/Shutterstock.com

pp.76–77 © View Apart/Shutterstock.com

pp.78–79 chess pieces © Plateresca/Shutterstock.com; playing cards © Eisfrei/Shutterstock.com; film-related images and book case © Julia August/Shutterstock.com; book © Maltiase/Shutterstock.com; sun © Katsiaryna Chumakova/Shutterstock.com; bike © Nancy White/Shutterstock.com

p.80 © Stefa_Stefo4ka/Shutterstock.com

p.81 © Eugenio Marongiu/Shutterstock.com

pp.82–83 houses © Motorama/Shutterstock.com; book and moon © davooda/Shutterstock.com; plants © Happy Art/Shutterstock.com; pen and paintbrush © Alexandr III/Shutterstock.com; yin-yang symbol, figures, teacup and candle © Marina Shevchenko/Shutterstock.com; kettle, cloud, sun and paw print © Anna_leni/Shutterstock.com

pp.84–85 background © Nailia Schwarz/Shutterstock.com; arrows © Lyudmyla Ishchenko/Shutterstock.com

pp.86–87, 88–89 (background) © ilolab/Shutterstock.com

pp.90–91 © Dmitry Zimin/Shutterstock.com

p.93 © Trum Ronnarong/Shutterstock.com

p.96 © Guzel Studio/Shutterstock.com

p.99 © JeniFoto/Shutterstock.com

p.101 © Natasha Breen/Shutterstock.com

p.103 © Vera Dimov/Shutterstock.com

p.105 © Maren Winter/Shutterstock.com

p.107 © DUSAN ZIDAR/Shutterstock.com

p.108 © Foxys Forest Manufacture/Shutterstock.com

p.110 © Natalia Hubbert/Shutterstock.com

p.113 pepper © alfaori/Shutterstock.com; pumpkin © Olga_Serova/Shutterstock.com; all other images © Calesh/Shutterstock.com

p.115 © leonori/Shutterstock.com

p.116 © Jenny Sturm/Shutterstock.com

p.117 © antalogiya/Shutterstock.com

pp.118–119 © jakkapan/Shutterstock.com

p.123 © Stock Rocket/Shutterstock.com

p.128 background © Tanya Syrytsyna/Shutterstock.com; illustrations © vectopicta/Shutterstock.com

p.129 book © JUN3/Shutterstock.com; light bulb and umbrella © Kseniia Bakshaeva/Shutterstock.com; text boxes and arrow © knahthra/Shutterstock.com

pp.130–131 book © JUN3/Shutterstock.com; cup and present © Kseniia Bakshaeva/Shutterstock.com; feather and diamond © vectopicta/Shutterstock.com; text boxes, question mark and arrow © knahthra/Shutterstock.com; Thursday © Luzik/Shutterstock.com

pp.136–137, 144–145 © Anastasia Panfilova/Shutterstock.com

pp.138–139 © Cat_arch_angel/Shutterstock.com

pp.140–141 ear © Rova N/Shutterstock.com; tree © Happy Art/Shutterstock.com; fruit © justone/Shutterstock.com; raindrop, hills and stones © Tom Devonald; all other images © Anna_leni/Shutterstock.com

p.142 © everst/Shutterstock.com

p.143 © TairA/Shutterstock.com

p.151 © Olga_Serova/Shutterstock.com

p.152 © Siberica/Shutterstock.com

p.153 © Nancy White/Shutterstock.com

pp.154–155 © Elizaveta Ruzanova/Shutterstock.com

pp.158–159 background © watercolor 15/Shutterstock.com

p.159 flowers © Stefa_Stefo4ka/Shutterstock.com